12/1

KT-382-278

BNKY

Please return/renew this item by the last date shown
on this label, or on your self-service receipt.

To renew this item, visit **www.librarieswest.org.uk**
or contact your library.

Your Borrower number and PIN are required.

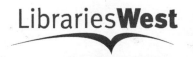

The Cancer
Prevention
Manual

The Cancer Prevention Manual

Simple rules to reduce the risks

SECOND EDITION

IAN OLVER
Professor of Translational Cancer Research
Director, Sansom Institute for Health Research
University of South Australia
Australia

FRED STEPHENS
Emeritus Professor, Department of Surgery
The University of Sydney
Australia

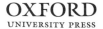

OXFORD
UNIVERSITY PRESS

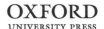

OXFORD
UNIVERSITY PRESS

Great Clarendon Street, Oxford, OX2 6DP,
United Kingdom

Oxford University Press is a department of the University of Oxford.
It furthers the University's objective of excellence in research, scholarship,
and education by publishing worldwide. Oxford is a registered trade mark of
Oxford University Press in the UK and in certain other countries

First Edition published in 2002
Second Edition published in 2016
Impression: 1

Published in the United States of America by Oxford University Press
198 Madison Avenue, New York, NY 10016, United States of America

British Library Cataloguing in Publication Data
Data available

Library of Congress Control Number: 2015938774

ISBN 978–0–19–871985–4

Printed in Great Britain by
Clays Ltd, St Ives plc

Dedication

Both of us dedicate this book to our families who are not only encouraging and supportive but have been very helpful in commenting on the various drafts and making suggestions which have improved the presentation.

We also acknowledge our gratitude to the many patients with cancer whom we treated, who served as encouragement to us to spread the cancer prevention message as widely as possible.

Preface

It is amazing just how much new information there is about cancer prevention and early detection since the first edition of this book 16 years ago. It has meant a complete rewrite, but keeping the aim of making it easily understood by the general public.

The incidence of cancer is increasing as more people live to an age when cancer is likely. The death rate from cancer is beginning to fall where better treatment is available and population screening for common cancers like breast, cervix, and bowel cancers allows early detection when the cancers are curable. More is known about the causes of cancer.

The changes in the text include de-emphasizing sections like breast self-examination, since mammographic screening better detects early cancer and pre-invasive cancer. We have added preventable risk factors such as alcohol consumption as well as including new information on, for example, vaccination against human papilloma virus and hepatitis B to prevent cervix and liver cancers. There are now three population screening programmes of proven efficacy where colorectal screening has been added to cervix and breast screening. More data on the risks and benefits of these programmes are available. There is also intriguing information on a possible role of aspirin in preventing bowel cancer in those at high risk. There is still little evidence that the potential benefit of population prostate screening justifies the harms but the place of PSA (prostate-specific antigen) testing is clearer. Although the data on cancer causation are equivocal, the public will want comments on mobile phones and airport scanners. Similar updates are needed where asbestos exposure applies not only to industry but home renovators.

The scope and the general character of the book remains similar to the first edition with a text written at the level of understanding of the general public and illustrated with line drawings. The technical terms are explained in the text rather than their meaning presented in a glossary. All of the information presented is based on the best evidence available.

Contents

1

What is cancer?

Introduction to cancer

Cancer is a disease where the normal cells of the body grow out of control. It is caused because several of the genes inside the cell which help control growth become altered (mutated). A diagram of a gene is shown in Figure 1.1. You can be born with some altered genes or acquire others when cells become exposed to agents in your environment which cause cancer, such as the chemicals in tobacco or radiation from the sun. Several gene mutations need to occur before a cell turns into a cancer cell by growing out of control. The process of developing cancer most often takes many years or even decades.

In the normal body, if you cut your finger, for example, the skin grows from each side until it covers the wound but then it stops. In other parts of the body, cells that become old are replaced with just as many cells as are needed. A cancer, however, keeps on growing, destroying the function of the organ in which it arises. What is more, cancer cells can break away and travel in the bloodstream or tiny vessels called lymphatics to distant organs of the body where they can grow and cause widespread damage as secondary cancers. It is like weeds being spread by the wind until they find a suitable soil in which to take root.

Cancer is actually over 200 different diseases since each organ or tissue in the body can give rise to its own cancer. Although the cancers each have the same underlying problem of cells growing out of control, they are all different. They are due to exposure to different cancer-causing agents in the environment or inherited gene defects, and they grow at different speeds. At the genetic level they have different patterns of altered genes. We now know that even cancers in the same organ can differ markedly in their patterns of altered genes. This will influence what treatments they will respond to. So although people speak of a 'cure' for cancer it is far more likely that different treatments will be needed for each type of cancer.

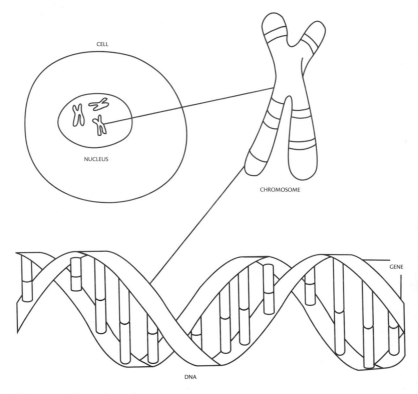

Figure 1.1 The nucleus of the cell contains DNA (deoxyribonucleic acid) in chromosomes that are further divided into genes.

Cancer by any other name . . .

It can be confusing that there are so many different words that are used for cancer. Originally cancer came from the Greek word for crab, *karkinos*. It was named because in some cancers there was a body and swollen blood vessels radiating out which looked like the legs of a crab. This is shown in Figure 1.2. This gives rise to the term *carcinoma* which is the name given to the cancers that arise from many of the body organs. The term *sarcoma* is used when cancer arises from supporting tissues like muscles or fat. You may hear the word *neoplasm* or *neoplastic* which really just refers to new growth of cells, which may be a cancer. Finally, you will encounter the word *tumour*. This just means 'lump' and not all lumps are cancerous. So-called benign tumours are not cancers because they grow locally in the tissue where they start but don't

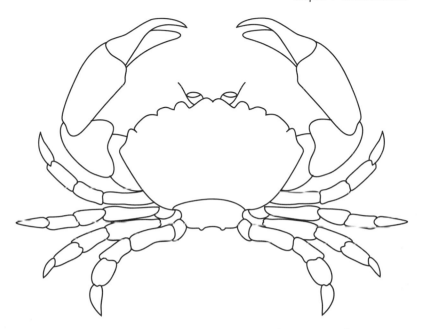

Figure 1.2 Cancer the crab, suggesting how cancer extends into surrounding tissues.

invade the organ around them or spread to other sites. They can cause local problems by putting pressure on surrounding cells but are usually slow growing. A *malignant* tumour is a cancer which invades the local organ as it grows and throws off cells into the bloodstream that can spread to distant sites. Sometimes the term malignancy is used when referring to cancer.

A couple of other common terms that we should introduce here are the words metastases and secondaries. These both refer to the cancer that has spread to other organs. A cancer is named by the organ in which it starts. Depending on the primary or original site of the cancer, the cells that spread have a preference to spread to different organs. Breast cancer, for example, when it spreads to distant organs, mainly goes to the liver, bones, lung, and brain. When that occurs it is still called breast cancer, and is not named by the site to which it spreads; so we refer to it as breast cancer in the liver, rather than liver cancer.

Treatment

Many cancers can remain in their site of origin or just spread locally to lymph nodes or glands which drain that site. When that is the case they may be able to be completely removed by surgery; alternatively the entire site of the primary cancer and also the local lymph nodes are covered by a radiotherapy field. These are therapies which are used to control localized cancer. When cancer spreads beyond its primary site it needs to be treated with therapies that will travel around the body in the bloodstream. These can be drugs (known as chemotherapy), hormone therapy, or immunotherapy.

For some cancers, the drug therapies are given after the local treatment has removed all the visible cancer because this has been found to prevent relapse. This so-called adjuvant therapy is presumed to be killing microscopic cells that have spread from the primary site before they can establish themselves as secondaries in other organs.

Know what prevents cancer

Cancer control involves a whole spectrum of activities including diagnosis and both anticancer treatments and supportive care measures to improve symptom control. People who survive cancer also require continuing support.

The focus of this book is on how cancer can be prevented. There are a number of lifestyle factors which can reduce the risk of cancer. With some cancers, for those at high risk of developing cancer, surgical removal of organs has been recommended or medication can be taken to prevent cancer. Examples include hormone therapy to prevent some breast cancers and aspirin in the case of bowel cancer. Individuals at high risk may also benefit from more intensive screening to either detect cancer early or, in the case of bowel or cervix cancer, detect and remove early changes before they develop into invasive cancer.

People make lifestyle choices for many reasons other than cancer risk, but everyone should at least be aware of what choices can change their chances of developing cancer and it is this information that we seek to spread.

2

What causes cancer?

The causes of cancer

We have said that cancer is a disease caused by genes functioning abnormally. The genetic material in the core of each cell, DNA (deoxyribonucleic acid), is divided into segments called genes. Each gene contains the instructions to make a protein which is needed for the body to function. Some proteins may determine hair colour, while others help control the growth of a cell and if they are changed or mutated this could increase your chance of getting cancer. For example, genes can act as tumour suppressor genes. They repair DNA and tell cells when to die. If these genes become mutated, the cells may grow out of control, leading to cancer.

Inherited gene mutations

Every cell in the body contains all of the genes. For a specialized cell, some of the genes won't be needed and are switched off. Mutation is the process of a change in one or more genes. There are two types of mutations: inherited and acquired. If a mutation is passed on by a parent through the egg or sperm then every cell of the new person will have it. If the mutation occurs after the egg and sperm have combined then it is called an acquired mutation and because it wasn't present in the egg or sperm it cannot be passed on to every new cell.

When we talk about inheriting a cancer we are really talking about inheriting a mutated gene which could trigger cancer. It is estimated that only 10% of cancers are inherited and 90% are acquired or sporadic. Even if you inherit a mutated gene you may not always get cancer, depending on other damage that needs to occur to other genes to trigger cancer. You receive one copy of a gene from each parent, and if one is mutated you will have to acquire a mutation in the other one before the gene stops working. For example, the BRCA1 (breast cancer 1) mutation involved in breast and ovarian cancer is associated with an 80% lifetime risk of developing breast cancer, not 100%. If you have inherited a mutated gene you have a 50% chance of passing it on to each of your children.

There are some features of inherited cancers which differentiate them from sporadic cancers. They occur at a younger age (because with sporadic cancer you would have to acquire mutations to both copies of a gene to knock out that gene's function and acquiring two mutations takes longer than starting with one and only having to acquire the second). This means that screening should start earlier for inherited than with sporadic cancers. Sometimes inherited mutations are associated with multiple cancers. The discovery of an inherited mutation in a person means that their blood relatives may also have the mutation.

Not all cancers that run in families are due to inherited genetic mutations. For example, a family of heavy smokers simply share the same acquired cancer risk factor. Apart from the younger age of onset, other features suggesting that a cancer arises from an inherited gene mutation are if the cancer is rare, if multiple cancers are diagnosed in the same person, if cancers occur in both of a pair of organs (e.g. both kidneys), or if cancer occurs in other than the usual sex (e.g. male breast cancer). The number of close relatives who have the same type of cancer is another clue.

It is beyond the scope of this manual to go into detail about types of inherited mutations, some of which are very rare; however, some examples will show the implications of being identified as having one of these.

Hereditary non-polyposis colorectal cancer

Hereditary non-polyposis colorectal cancer (HNPCC) or Lynch syndrome carries a high risk of bowel cancer which presents earlier than sporadic bowel cancers, often before the age of 50 years. The name is not completely accurate in that these people can have some polyps, just not the hundreds seen with another inherited condition, familial adenomatous polyposis.

Large bowel cancer is one of many cancers associated with HNPCC which includes cancers of the endometrium, ovary, small bowel, stomach, pancreas, bile duct, kidney, and brain. It can be associated with mutations in a number of genes responsible for DNA repair. These can be tested for, or a piece of a cancer tested for changes called microsatellite instability due to the genetic mutation. If this is present it suggests HNPCC.

The implication is that parents, brothers and sisters, and children of a person found to have HNPCC have a 50% chance of having it themselves and should be offered testing. If positive they should be screened early for bowel cancer and other cancers where testing is available.

Hereditary breast and ovarian cancer syndrome

Hereditary breast and ovarian cancer syndrome (HBOCS) has the feature of an inherited mutation condition in that the cancers present earlier than most, often in both breasts and sometimes with ovarian cancer. A couple of the main gene mutations responsible were eventually discovered, in the *BRCA1* and *BRCA2* genes, but there are more genes still to be identified. Other cancers that have been associated with mutations in *BRCA1* or *BRCA2* are fallopian tube cancer, primary peritoneal cancer, male breast cancer, pancreatic cancer, and prostate cancer, the last three more often with *BRCA2* mutations.

Again, close relatives have a 50% chance of also having the mutation and people will be selected by genetic counsellors for testing based on the likelihood of HBOCS being present according to the history of the breast cancer in the patient and the family history. There are difficult decisions to make for those carrying one of the mutations. They will have up to an 80% lifetime risk of cancer but this means some people may be old before the cancer develops. The most aggressive option is bilateral mastectomy and oophorectomy (removing the ovaries) to reduce the risk. Earlier and intense screening is a second option and there may be hormonal medication that can be taken to reduce the risk.

Li Fraumeni syndrome

This is an example of a rare syndrome which can cause multiple less common cancers, which start in childhood and where each person can develop multiple cancers. It is caused by a mutation in a tumour suppressor gene. The cancers include sarcomas (cancers of supporting tissue like muscles or bones), leukaemias, brain tumours, adrenal tumours, and breast cancer. There may be little to do to prevent many of these cancers but this syndrome does make people more sensitive to developing cancer after radiation and this may dictate treatment choices.

Sporadic cancers

Most cancers are sporadic and arise because of exposure to the environment in which we live. Some causes of cancer are shown in Figure 2.1. It takes several mutations of genes to trigger cancer; how many may differ between cancers. How agents in the environment can trigger cancer is being explored as part of the field of epigenetics.

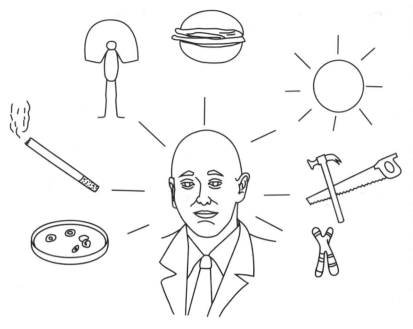

Figure 2.1 Think about the many causes of cancer.

Epigenetics

Epigenetic changes are heritable changes in the expression of genes (that is, whether they produce their protein product) which occur without the structure of the DNA (that is, the sequence of its component bases) itself being altered. The common alterations are that the DNA undergoes a chemical change (methylation) that can switch off tumour suppressor genes or DNA repair genes and proteins called histones, around which DNA wraps itself, can be modified and this affects whether the message carried by the gene can be transcribed. This could result in cancer if a tumour suppressor gene was silenced in this way.

Epigenetic changes may be involved in the progression of a cancer, perhaps by enhancing the possibility that it will spread. They can be involved in directly initiating a cancer or priming a cell to promote it becoming cancerous when exposed to a subsequent trigger for DNA mutation. The study of the changes in these proteins gives us new mechanisms for how drugs and agents in the environment can promote cancer by interacting with them. So, various diets, for example, may provide methyl groups for DNA methylation while agents like arsenic and cadmium certainly can change methylation.

Environmental exposures causing cancer

Having explored the mechanism for agents influencing the genetic material in a cell to trigger cancer, we now need to touch on the range of agents which have been implicated in causing cancer. We will explore some in more detail when we explore options for preventing cancer.

Tobacco

As a preventable cause of cancer tobacco tops most lists. Tobacco smoke contains over 4000 chemicals, at least 70 of which are well documented to cause cancer. Nicotine in cigarettes is highly addictive. There are the same constituents in cigars as in cigarettes and even being exposed to second-hand smoke from someone else smoking nearby increases your cancer risk. Smokeless tobacco can cause cancer through the nitrosamines it contains and this particularly affects the head and neck, oesophagus, and pancreas. There is now a growing trend for electronic cigarettes (e-cigarettes) that don't contain tobacco but instead heat a fluid containing flavourings and sometimes nicotine. Most of the chemicals being inhaled have not been tested and the risk of cancer associated with them not adequately explored. Certainly for those e-cigarettes containing nicotine it may be just another way to addict people to nicotine.

Diet and physical activity

This is second to tobacco as a risk factor as the Western diet is associated with an increasingly obese community. In general, we eat too much fat and processed food and insufficient fresh fruit and vegetables. Red meat, particularly if barbecued rather than slow grilled, and processed meats increase cancer risk. Diet, lack of exercise, and sedentary workplaces all have independent impacts on cancer. Alcohol is a major carcinogen where the risk of cancer starts at zero (but two standard drinks per day is considered reasonably safe).

Sun and ultraviolet (UV) radiation

The very high incidence of skin cancer makes the burden of skin cancer the highest of all cancers, and yet both melanomas and non-melanomas are largely preventable by reducing harmful exposure to UV radiation from the sun or solariums.

Radiation exposure

Much of what we know about cancers related to high-energy (often called ionizing) radiation comes from exposure to nuclear weapons and nuclear power plant accidents. Therapeutic and diagnostic radiation may pose a risk depending on the dose. Radon is a naturally occurring source of radiation in rock and soil and can be harmful with continuous exposure if homes are built in these areas.

Radiofrequency radiation is low dose and around us in the atmosphere at low levels all of the time. Man-made sources include radio and television signals, mobile phones and phone towers, radar, Wi-Fi and Bluetooth, microwave ovens, and whole-body security scanners. Although there is the possibility of risk, to date no studies have demonstrated an actual association with cancer, and the possible mechanism for such low-level radiation causing cancer is undetermined.

Extremely low-frequency radiation (ELF) may be generated next to power lines or electrical devices including computer and television screens. There are no consistent studies which link this type of radiation to cancer in adults and there is limited but conflicting evidence about childhood leukaemia in children living close to power lines.

Infections

Whilst a number of infectious agents are linked to cancer, in general you can't 'catch' cancer by casual contact with a person with cancer. Examples of viruses linked to cancer include HIV (human immunodeficiency virus) which causes AIDS and predisposes to cancers like anal cancer and lymphoma; HPV (human papilloma virus) and cancer of the cervix; the Epstein–Barr virus and nasopharyngeal cancer and lymphoma; hepatitis B and C viruses and liver cancer; HHV-8 (human herpes virus 8 which is associated with Kaposi's sarcoma); HTLV-1 (human T-lymphotropic virus 1) linked to a rare T-cell lymphoma and MCV (Merkel cell polyomavirus) which causes an aggressive skin cancer called Merkel cell carcinoma.

Bacteria linked to cancer include *Helicobacter pylori* and stomach cancer. *Chlamydia trachomatis* is a sexually transmitted bacterium which may help promote cancer of the cervix in association with HPV. There are also some parasitic worms like *Clonorchis sinensis*, a liver fluke often acquired by eating raw fish and linked to bile duct cancer, and *Schistosoma haematobium*, which is a parasite found in water in South East Asia, the Middle East, and Africa which can cause bladder cancer.

Occupational exposures

There are many industrial processes which can lead to exposure to hazardous substances. They include asbestos which can lead to mesothelioma and lung cancer; benzene associated with lymphomas; hair dyes with lymphoma;

arsenic with bladder cancer and lymphomas; vinyl chlorides with angiosarco-mas of the liver; fertilizers and pesticides with lymphoma; nickel and crystal-line silica with lung cancer, and many more chemicals that have the potential to cause cancer if the exposure is of a sufficient amount.

Pollution

We are sure that inhaling polluted air in our big cities is not good for people, but it has been difficult to pick out specific agents from the vast number that we are exposed to which can be shown to cause cancer. Exposure to diesel exhaust is coming under scrutiny and can be associated with developing blad-der cancer.

Medical therapies

Treating cancer with radiotherapy and chemotherapy rarely can lead to sec-ond cancers which occur years later. Children who have multiple CT (com-puted tomography) scans have a higher risk of leukaemia and brain tumours. Exposure to diethylstilboestrol caused breast cancers in women who received it to prevent spontaneous abortion, and their daughters developed breast can-cer and clear cell cancers of the vagina and cervix. Using hormone replace-ment therapy can predispose to breast cancer, oral contraceptive therapy can predispose to cancer of the cervix, and tamoxifen to endometrial cancer. Growth hormones used in orthopaedics may predispose to sarcoma.

Cancer statistics

The incidence of most cancers increases with age as genetic errors become more common, and so as our population survives to greater ages, the inci-dence of cancer will increase. Added to this is the increased incidence expected as the Western population becomes more obese. The good news in Western populations is that there has been a decline in cancer deaths, attributed to screening, early detection, and improved treatments.

The International Agency for Research on Cancer keeps the Globocan data-base of cancer statistics (see Bibliography). There were 14.1 million cases of cancer diagnosed around the world in 2012, 7.4 million cases in men and 6.7 million in women, and this is expected to increase to 24 million by 2035.

Excluding non-melanoma skin cancer, lung, female breast, colorectal, and stomach cancer represent 40% of all cancers diagnosed around the world. There were 8.2 million deaths due to cancer around the world in 2012. The prevalence of cancer, that is, all the people surviving cancer in the previous 5 years, was 32.5 million people.

Countries classified as low or medium development nations had 44% of the cancer incidence and 53% of the deaths. In 2008, it was estimated that a staggering 163.9 million years of healthy life were lost globally to cancer. This reinforces the need to identify the modifiable risk factors and the exposure to them.

3

Lifestyle changes that prevent cancer

Modifiable risk factors for cancer

You can't choose your family and the gene mutations you may inherit which will predispose you towards developing cancer. However, there are modifiable risk factors related to lifestyle that you can control and this chapter aims to tell you what they are. It is estimated that a third of cancer deaths could be prevented by modifying lifestyle factors alone. That's quite impressive. We are going to cover the major factors such as stopping smoking tobacco, controlling your weight, including the impact of modifying diet and alcohol consumption, doing more exercise, and protecting yourself from the sun.

We will look at the cancer hazards which may be in the workplace and will discuss other possibilities that are often raised such as the use of mobile phones, airport scanners, stress, and depression. We then examine screening and early detection and finally which cancers could be prevented through vaccination.

Smoking

There is nothing more effective that we can do to prevent cancer than not to smoke. This is still the case even though Australia's adult daily smoking rate was down to 12.8% by 2014. Did you know that smoking contributes to a fifth of our cancer burden and is linked to 16 different types of cancer, not only lung cancer? Smoking also causes almost as many deaths from heart and vascular disease, including stroke, as it does from cancer, not to mention the burden of chronic lung disease. Two of every three people who smoke will die of smoking-related disease and the life expectancy of smokers is around 10 years less than non-smokers. This is shown in Figure 3.1. That should be enough reason never to start, or at least to quit.

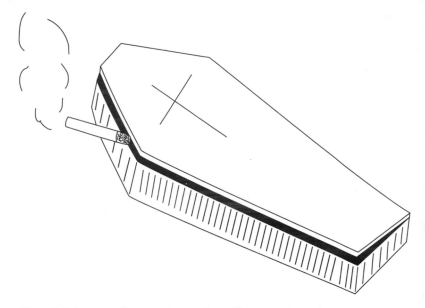

Figure 3.1 Do you really want 10 years of your life to go up in smoke?

Smoking and cancers

In addition to lung cancer, other main cancers caused by smoking are those affecting the throat, particularly in smokers who drink alcohol, as well as bladder and kidney cancer. Unfortunately, in addition to the smoker, others exposed to the second-hand smoke exhaled by smokers are at risk of the same diseases, particularly if someone smokes in the home. Children are vulnerable and it can also affect the babies of women exposed during pregnancy.

Around eight in every ten smokers became addicted as teenagers. That is why it is so important that adult role models set a good example, advertising is banned so it can no longer show smoking as 'cool', and cigarette packs are made plain to reduce the lure of attractive packaging. It is a myth that you can just try it and give up at any time, because the nicotine in cigarettes causes a powerful addition that can make quitting very difficult. The message is DON'T START SMOKING!

Ways to quit

We know it can be hard to quit but help is available and there are many ways to quit. You should find one that is suited to you. Telephone quit-lines provide support and information or you can talk to your GP. A good way to start to quit is to try to quit on your own ('cold turkey') and simply throw away the current pack and don't buy another. This appears to be more effective than trying to gradually reduce the number smoked, unless as part of a comprehensive programme. Certainly trying to wean off smoking by changing to a low-tar cigarette has not been found to be effective. There are self-help booklets that will guide you in how to stop smoking and stay that way. The important thing is not to become discouraged if the first quit attempt doesn't last, but to simply start again. The more attempts that you make take you closer to success.

If you need more help, there are courses available that offer support and have a high success rate. These courses vary in quality and you should be wary of courses that make extravagant claims.

If courses or counselling are not effective you may wish to try medication to reduce the cravings of the addiction during the quit attempt. The most common are nicotine replacement therapies which come in many types including tablets and lozenges, gums, mouth sprays, skin patches, and inhalers. There are other prescription drugs, such as bupropion, which should be commenced with medical supervision.

Some people want to try other techniques such as hypnotherapy, herbs, or acupuncture. They are not routinely recommended because proof of their effectiveness is thin. Likewise, some are advocating the use of e-cigarettes for help with quitting but we need further proof of their efficacy, and for non-smokers they could just be another way of becoming addicted to nicotine.

The banning of advertising has been effective in reducing the temptation to smoke. This includes plain packaging so that the packaging can't be used to tempt young people to take up the habit. Mass media campaigns show the damage to your health of smoking. With the price of cigarettes rising sharply as governments use price increases to encourage quitting, you will save money by not smoking. It is often good to reward yourself with a holiday or a gift to celebrate your success.

Most recently e-cigarettes have appeared. These are devices often made to look like cigarettes but are battery-powered vaporizers which produce a mist rather than tobacco smoke. This fluid can contain nicotine, propylene glycol, glycerine, and flavourings which are then in the vapour. It is meant to create a similar feel to cigarette smoking. It is promoted as being safer than cigarettes because of the absence of tobacco and a possible method of weaning smokers off cigarettes, although there are already many nicotine replacement products available.

However, there is only emerging research which has not yet answered the question of whether e-cigarettes will aid quitting or simply attract young people, who then move on to cigarettes. There has not been much research on the safety of the chemicals in the vapour. Until there is more information, why do we need yet another way to addict people to nicotine?

Health benefits of quitting

The benefits to your health from quitting begin almost immediately as the body begins to repair itself. Within just 6 hours your heart rate will slow and blood pressure will decrease. Within the first day you have got rid of almost all the nicotine, and the carbon monoxide in your blood drops sharply to allow more oxygen into your body.

In the first week the lungs are better able to clear the dust and mucous and your sense of taste and smell will start to recover. Within the first couple of months you will notice that you are not coughing and wheezing as much, you are less prone to infection, and the blood flow to your hands and feet has improved.

After a year your risk of heart attack and stroke will have dropped. By 10 years your risk of lung cancer will have halved and will continue to drop. By 15 years you have a similar risk of heart disease as a non-smoker. So don't delay, get started!

Diet, exercise, and obesity

'You are what you eat.' This phrase, with its origins in the 1800s, is quite unfortunate for a population today that is becoming increasingly obese. When we think about being overweight and health we think more about diabetes or heart disease. However, it is estimated that one-quarter of all cancers could be prevented through good food choices and adequate exercise. If we had a drug that promised such an outcome everyone would be clamouring for it. Although being overweight or obese, and its underlying causes of an unhealthy diet and lack of exercise are independent risk factors for cancer, together they are second only to smoking tobacco as preventable factors. This is shown in Figure 3.2.

Diet

Although the headlines often scream at us about specific foods, be it pomegranates for prostate cancer or broccoli for breast cancer, usually these are based on very small studies which may be unreliable. Often the best we can

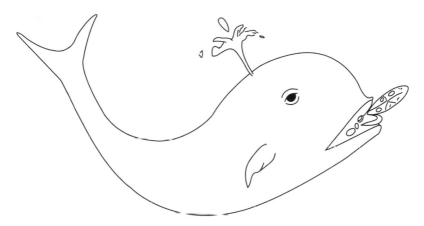

Figure 3.2 A whale of a time overeating may reduce your time living.

do from large studies across populations is to make general recommendations about food groups. Most are common sense. A diet which favours fresh fruit and vegetables over fatty processed foods is likely to be much healthier.

It is known that unhealthy eating increases your cancer risk but healthy eating can protect against cancer. For example there is evidence that increasing consumption of processed meats may increase the risk of bowel cancer while foods containing dietary fibre decrease the risk of bowel cancer.

What are we eating? A large nutrition and physical activity survey of Australians found that although three-quarters of them reported eating vegetables, less than 7% consumed the recommended intake of five servings each day. The individuals least likely to eat vegetables were young adults (19–30 years old) and the most likely were 4- to 8-year-olds! 'Eat your greens, Billie, and you'll grow up nice and strong.'

Fruit consumption was better, with over half of the population eating at least two servings of fruit each day. Men, however, lagged behind women. The big problem, though, is that we are getting almost a third of our energy from eating fats, which is considered far too high. So let's look now at specific foods; but remember what you eat is all about balance. It is rarely about all or none, but more about not having too much of some foods and too little of others. It is also important to know the well-established links between cancer and food and beverages. There is no point arguing over whether green tea is associated with a small reduction in cancer risk whilst ignoring a major risk like alcohol consumption!

Meat

What do we mean when we talk about meat? There are the red meats like beef, veal, pork, mutton, and lamb. Then there are what are often termed white meats like fish and poultry. Finally there are the processed or preserved meats which have other additives and include smoked, salted, or cured meats like bacon, ham and salami, sausages, and canned meat.

It is processed meat that most convincingly has been associated with an increased risk of developing bowel cancer. As the quantity of red meat consumed goes up, so does the risk of bowel cancer. There is less convincing evidence of an association of both red meat and processed meat with oesophageal and lung cancer, processed meats with prostate cancer and stomach cancer, and red meat with pancreatic and endometrial (lining of the uterus or womb) cancer. However, to make the point that we are not suggesting an all-or-nothing approach as we would with smoking, for example, lean red meat is an important source of iron in the diet as well as zinc, vitamin B_{12} and protein.

On the positive side, for meats, there is limited evidence suggesting that fish may reduce the risk of breast, bowel, and prostate cancer. Fish contains omega-3 polyunsaturated fats which may protect against cancer.

The difficulty of being precise about meats causing cancer can be illustrated by looking at how they may do this. There are several possibilities. Meats that are preserved have a high concentration of chemicals (N-nitroso compounds) which can be converted by bacteria in the gut into cancer-causing chemicals. Red meat also has lower amounts of these, whereas they are not found in fish or chicken. However, that is not the only explanation. The ability to cause cancer may relate also to the fat content of the meat. Then, there are differences in the likelihood of cancer which are related to how the meat is cooked. It should come as no surprise that if you barbeque meat to look like a burnt offering, this produces cancer-causing chemicals which are not produced by slow-cooking or grilling meat. Of course, how healthy a meal is will depend on what accompanies the meat. Vegetables, fruit, and wholegrain cereals help ensure a healthy balance.

Putting all of this information together from a cancer prevention viewpoint, we can recommend that you limit your lean red meat intake to no more than three or four servings each week. The amount of each serving should be about 65–100 grams, which is about half a cup of mince, two slices of roast meat, or two small chops. It is better if meat is slowly grilled, casseroled, or microwaved rather than barbequing or cooking at high temperature by frying or grilling.

Processed or preserved meats like salami, bacon, ham, and various sausages should be eaten only occasionally or avoided all together. Often those meats are also high in salt and fat which are unhealthy if consumed in large amounts. You are encouraged to eat fish, particularly oily fish, at least twice each week.

Omega-3 fatty acids and fish

Omega-3 fatty acids are found in oily fish such as swordfish, Atlantic salmon, Spanish mackerel, gemfish, and oysters. They are found in some oils such as canola, soybean, linseed, and walnut. Fish may reduce the chance of breast and prostate cancer while increasing the amount of omega-3 fatty acids may reduce breast cancer risk. They work by blocking the triggering of cancer or interfering with oestrogen, a female hormone that can stimulate breast cancer.

We suggest that you eat a couple of fish meals each week and in addition some of the oils high in omega-3 fatty acids.

Salt

Salt is used for flavouring and preserving foods. You may be aware that eating a lot of salt can cause high blood pressure and heart disease, but it has also been linked to developing stomach cancer.

One source of salt is what you add to food at the table or while cooking, but perhaps more of a trap is just how much salt can be part of processed or pack-aged foods. You may be surprised if you read the nutrition information panel on the back of food packages just how much sodium (salt is sodium chloride) that some foods contain. A rule of thumb is to aim for foods where the salt content is listed at no more than 120 milligrams per 100 grams since this is considered a low-salt food.

Some of the high-salt foods are sauces such as soy and fish sauce, stock cubes, soups, cereals, and bread. There is also often a great variation in salt content between different brands of the same foods, so it is worth checking the panel at the back of the packaging or front of pack labels, where they exist, which summarize the main nutritional content of foods.

You should generally aim for no more than 1½ teaspoons of salt each day (2300 milligrams of sodium, which is 6 grams of salt). This may be achieved by not adding salt and avoiding processed foods with a high salt content.

Wholegrain cereals and dietary fibre

If you want to increase the dietary fibre in your diet you would increase your consumption of wholegrain cereals, vegetables, seeds, nuts, and legumes such as lentils, peas, and beans. Foods high in fibre include wheat bran and oat bran, seeds such as sunflower seeds, nuts, particularly raw almonds, and wholemeal breads.

In addition to decreasing the risk of type 2 diabetes and heart disease, there is convincing evidence that eating these foods decreases the chance of developing bowel cancer and may also lower the risk of oesophageal cancer. There are several possible ways that fibre can work to reduce cancer risk. Increasing the bulk of the stool will decrease the time it needs to pass through the bowel and therefore the exposure of the bowel wall to cancer-causing chemicals.

There are also direct effects of fibre on chemicals that can cause cancer. The other major effect of foods with fibre is that they are low fat and control energy intake and appetite. They therefore help control weight and obesity, which is linked to an increased risk of cancers, including of the endometrium (lining of the womb), kidney, breast (in women after menopause), bowel, oesophagus, and pancreas.

How much of these fibre-rich foods should be eaten each day? The technical answer is about 25 grams of dietary fibre for women and 30 grams for men. That translates to two servings of wholegrain foods, two servings of fruit, and five servings of vegetables. A 'serving' means two slices of wholegrain bread or 1⅓ cups of breakfast cereal. For fruit, examples of a serving are a medium-sized apple or orange, or two small apricots, whilst a ½ cup of cooked vegetables or lentils is considered a single serving.

Fruit and vegetables

Fruit and vegetables are likely to protect against some cancers because they contain nutrients which are known to have cancer protective effects. They contain fibre, but they also contain vitamins, minerals, and antioxidants, which are chemicals that protect against developing cancer. Plants also contain so-called phytochemicals, such as carotenoids and flavonoids, and it is likely that the combination of all of these give fruit and vegetables their anti-cancer properties. In addition, eating fruit and non-starchy vegetables (so we are not talking about potato chips!) instead of high-energy food with fats and carbohydrates, helps you control your weight. There is strong evidence that non-starchy vegetables and fruit protect against cancers of the mouth, throat, oesophagus, and stomach with less evidence about bowel, ovarian, and endometrial cancers. Fruit probably protects against lung cancer and garlic against bowel cancer and may also protect against pancreatic and liver cancers. In general, fruit and vegetables may not protect against prostate cancer except for foods containing lycopene, like tomatoes.

We recommend the 5 + 2 rule of thumb. Aim for five servings of vegetables and two servings of fruit each day and eat a variety of fruit and vegetables. Fresh produce with a mix of cooked and raw is ideal. It is important to note that the vitamins and antioxidants are much better consumed as whole fruit and vegetables than as supplements. The other question often raised is about 'organic' foods which are produced without added chemicals like pesticides, fertilizers, and hormones. Studies have not been done to show whether these have any greater impact on cancer, so their use is just a matter of individual choice. It would be wise, however, to wash or peel all fruits and vegetables before eating them.

Dairy foods

Dairy foods are the major source of calcium in the diet which is essential for the health of your bones and teeth. They also provide protein, vitamins, and minerals. From the cancer viewpoint, there is evidence that milk and calcium are protective against bowel cancer and possibly bladder cancer. It is not all good news, however, because studies also suggest that milk and dairy products and diets high in calcium may increase the risk of prostate cancer, and cheese may increase the risk of cancer of the lower large bowel.

Overall, the health benefits of dairy (particularly low-fat products) outweigh the risk and, as part of a varied diet, three servings of dairy, be it milk, cheese, or yoghurt, each day is what is usually recommended.

Sugary drinks

Many soft drinks are sweetened with sugar and have a very high sugar content. Whilst these drinks are not known to cause cancer in their own right, drinking them causes an increase in energy intake, leading to weight gain. We know that being overweight or obese contributes to cancer risk and so we discourage regular consumption of these drinks.

Changing dietary patterns

Population studies show that in countries that are mainly vegetarian and where meat products are not part of their standard diet, breast cancer is not a major problem in women and prostate cancer is not a major problem in men. When people from these countries migrate to countries with a standard Western meat-eating diet and they adopt the local non-vegetarian meat-eating diet the incidence of breast cancer in women and prostate cancer in men becomes similar to those who have always lived on traditional Western diets. This was particularly observed in people who migrated from Asian Countries to Hawaii and the United States.

The plant oestrogens and male hormones in soy and other plant foods have a significantly weaker hormonal effect than those in animal flesh. Studies continue as to whether the addition of plant hormones to people having a Western diet might reduce the incidence of breast cancer in women or prostate cancer in men.

Nutrients and supplements

It is fair to say that although some nutrients are available as supplements, it is better that they are consumed as part of the foods that contain them. This is how the body is used to seeing them. A good example of this is beta-carotene. This nutrient is found in vegetables or fruits, particularly those which are red or yellow like carrots, pumpkin, tomatoes, and apricots. It is converted in the body to vitamin A. It has been found that eating foods rich in beta-carotene will reduce your risk of lung, head and neck cancers, and maybe cancer of the oesophagus. However, in people who smoke, if beta-carotene is taken as a supplement as opposed to eating it in food, the risk of developing lung cancer seems to increase!

There is a similar situation with folate, which is a form of vitamin B. It is found in wholemeal bread and green leafed vegetables like broccoli, cabbage, and lettuce. Wheat flour in Australia is fortified with folic acid which plays an important part in reducing birth defects. Also eating foods high in folic acid probably reduces the risk of developing pancreatic cancer and may reduce the chances of getting oesophageal cancer, bowel cancer, and breast cancer after menopause in women with a family history. However, taking high doses of folate as supplements may stimulate polyps and cause early bowel cancers to progress.

The mineral selenium is found in soil and in varying amounts in Brazil nuts, fish and seafood, poultry, liver, meat, and cereals. Based on studies of large populations, where people who lived in regions where the soil contained more selenium had less cancer, trials of using supplements of selenium were undertaken. These tended to show the opposite effects where supplements of selenium or supplements of vitamin E tended to be associated with a greater risk of prostate cancer. Therefore neither selenium supplements can be recommended nor the health claims on foods containing selenium supported.

Exercise

Physical activity itself reduces the chances of developing some cancers. It also contributes to weight loss which in turn reduces the risk of a range of cancers. Being physically inactive is second only to tobacco in the lifestyle factors contributing to the burden of cancer in the community, being responsible for between 5% and 6% of that burden.

International estimates suggest that 14% of large bowel cancer and 11% of breast cancer after menopause is attributable to physical inactivity. If you compare the rate of bowel cancer among the most physically active people with the least physically active, there is a 40% reduction in bowel cancer in the most active. With breast cancer there is between a 20% and 40% reduction in the cancer risk by having regular exercise. Some studies have shown a 6% decrease in the risk of breast cancer for every additional hour of exercise each week. Exercise is also thought to protect against endometrial cancer and cancer of the ovary.

If you already have cancer, exercise is of benefit before, during, and after your treatment. It also can improve survival. It reduces the chance of the cancer returning in people who have been treated for bowel or breast cancer.

Although, in general, the cancer risk is improved as the amount of exercise increases, how much exercise should you try for? The greatest reduction in risk occurs between 30 to 60 minutes each day of moderate to intense exercise. Moderate exercise causes a noticeable increase in your heart rate and breathing and may occur with a brisk walk, gardening, doing slow laps swimming, and medium-paced cycling. Intense or vigorous exercise makes you quite breathless and includes running, fast cycling or rowing, and sports such as football, or netball, or doing aerobic workouts. Sporting choices are shown in Figure 3.3.

We would recommend at least 60 minutes of moderate exercise a day, but you should work towards 30 minutes of vigorous exercise. You should know that you don't have to do it all at once but can break it into 10-minute sessions and still derive the same benefit. That will often make it easier for you to reach your exercise quota during the course of a day. Whether you get more benefit from exercise when you are older or younger is yet to be determined.

The other side of the coin here is sedentary behaviour. When you are sedentary for long periods, irrespective of how much overall physical activity you do, you have an increased risk of bowel, endometrial, ovarian, and prostate cancer and in women there is an overall increase of dying of cancer. These days, sedentary behaviour can be part of your work life if you spend the day sitting at a desk using a computer or similarly as part of recreation, watching television, or playing computer games. You should try to look for times when you can be more active, such as using stairs instead of the lift. At work it may be worth exploring regular exercise breaks or the use of adjustable desks where you can

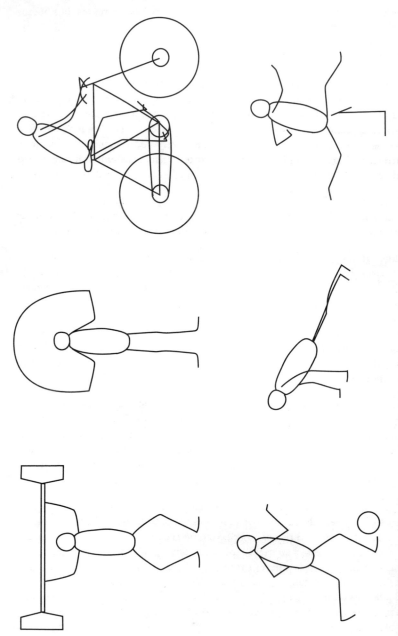

Figure 3.3 Exercise helps prevent cancer—but only if you start!

stand for periods of time. For recreation, spending some time doing physical exercise is important.

Obesity

There is now strong evidence that some cancers are linked to being overweight and obese. It is estimated that being overweight or obese accounts for around 4 in every 100 cancers and causes 14% of cancer deaths in men and 20% in women.

Most people gain weight because they take in more energy from what they eat and drink than they expend each day in exercise. Excess energy is mostly stored in the body as fat.

Commonly used measurements to assess obesity are the body mass index (BMI) and the waist circumference. You can calculate your BMI by dividing your weight in kilograms by your height in metres squared (height multiplied by itself). Obesity is defined as having a BMI of 30 or over and being overweight is a value between 25 and 30. Normal is from 18.5 to 25. The waist circumference is measured at the narrowest point for women and at the level of the navel for men. Women should have a waist circumference under 80 centimetres and men under 94 centimetres.

The distribution of the excess body fat is important. It is abdominal fat, as assessed by waist circumference, which increases cancer risk compared to fat elsewhere. Abdominal fat has been linked to bowel cancer, breast cancer after the menopause, and cancers of the pancreas and endometrium. The most convincing associations between body fat and cancer have been with large bowel cancer, breast cancer after the menopause, and cancers of the kidney, pancreas, oesophagus, and endometrium. There is probably also a link with ovarian and gall bladder cancer and maybe liver cancer. Strangely some studies suggest that excess fat before the menopause may decrease the risk of breast cancer.

As discussed, the causes of obesity (when you look at our whole population) are diet with excess energy (kilojoules) from energy-dense foods which are poor in nutrients and high in fat and sugar (often termed junk food), and a lack of expending energy particularly through exercise. In turn, the behaviours that lead to obesity can depend on the environment in which people live, and personal factors. Obesity is more common in people with lower incomes, and those who live more remotely, and in certain cultural groups such as people with Southern European and Middle Eastern backgrounds and indigenous Australians.

Home and school environments and exposure to heavy marketing of junk food can also influence food choices. It is important to establish healthy eating patterns in young people because between 25% and 50% of obese adolescents become obese adults. What is served in school tuck shops and eaten at home is influential on eating patterns.

The environment also includes where you live and whether you have access to safe parks or bicycle trails and places to walk and have public transport available rather than a car, all of which facilitate exercising. You also have to have accurate information available.

Government policy in supporting marketing campaigns for healthy eating and exercise and perhaps discouraging junk food advertising to children are also part of the environment in which you and your family make lifestyle choices. For example, clear food labelling which allows you to easily assess the sugar, fat, and salt content of packaged foods and to compare foods would seem important in enabling you to make healthy choices.

So, what to do about being overweight is clear. You should maintain a healthy body weight with a BMI of between 18.5 and 25 by increasing physical activity to at least 60 minutes of moderate exercise each day and eating according to energy needs. This often means having more fresh fruit, vegetables, cereals, and other low-fat foods in the diet instead of fatty and processed foods, and ensuring that your portion sizes at each meal are moderate. There is evidence that breastfeeding for at least 6 months helps prevent infants from becoming overweight or obese.

While the evidence that increased body weight and fat increases the risk of developing cancer there is less evidence about what happens to the cancer risk as we lose weight. There is some indication that if you are overweight and lose weight you lower your risk of breast cancer. For those of you who have cancer there is reasonable evidence from large studies that you will benefit from weight control and exercise which will improve your quality of life, decrease chances of the cancer returning, and improve your life expectancy.

Alcohol

It may be surprising or even distressing to some that something as commonly consumed as alcohol increases the risk of cancer. However, up to 6 in each 100 cancers can be attributed to long-term alcohol use. Alcohol has been associated with developing cancers of the throat and oesophagus, particularly when a person also smokes tobacco. It may be no surprise that it is also associated with cancer of the liver and this is even more likely in the presence of hepatitis B infection. However, it was the finding that it was part of the cause of common cancers (breast cancer in women and bowel cancer in men) that made it important to highlight the association. It is a lifestyle factor which can be modified.

The International Agency for Research on Cancer, which collects all of the world's data on what causes cancer, has reported the link between alcohol and cancer as definite. There is no safe level where cancer is concerned. The more that is consumed over the years, the greater the risk of developing cancer. It doesn't matter what type of alcohol you drink—beer, wine, or spirits: it is the overall amount of alcohol that is important.

Alcohol also contributes to weight gain, which is also a risk factor for bowel and breast cancers, as well as cancers of the oesophagus, pancreas, uterus, and kidney. This is particularly so when alcohol is added to a regular diet without compensating for the additional calories.

In Australia, almost one in five adults consume more alcohol over their life-time than is recommended. This includes older teenagers, but a national sur-vey in 2013 showed that the age of first drinking had increased to 15.7 years from 14.4 in 1998, which is encouraging. For the indigenous population, about one in six were consuming more than the recommended maximum of two standard drinks per day.

Are there any benefits to consuming alcohol? Some small studies suggest a decreased risk of cancer of the pancreas, but this is overwhelmed by the increased risk of other cancers. There are also some studies which suggest that low-level alcohol use may be beneficial to the heart, particularly drinking red wine. Other large trials have not been convincing on this finding and no major heart foundation has come out recommending alcohol for heart health.

What is a reasonable level of consumption? The National Health and Medical Research Council recommend that at no more than two standard drinks each day, the health risks are low. This seems reasonable although those who do not currently drink alcohol would be advised not to start. Of course you should know what a 'standard drink' means. A standard drink is 100 mL of red wine (13% alc. vol.) or a 375 mL can or bottle of mid-strength beer (3.5% alc. vol.). A 30 mL nip of spirits (40% alc. vol.) is also a standard drink. Furthermore, it is not always easy to judge because most wine glasses in restaurants would contain 150 mL. This is shown in Figure 3.4.

There is less publicity about alcohol and cancer and we don't see the health warnings that we see with other products. There is an advertising code that

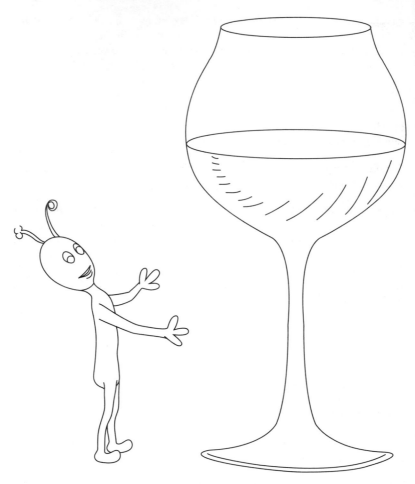

Figure 3.4 On what planet is that a standard drink?

if enforced would protect children from advertisements depicting alcohol as desirable when linked to sport, for example. GPs are encouraged to ask their patients about their alcohol consumption from about their mid-teens since inappropriate patterns of alcohol consumption in young people will certainly impact on their chances of chronic diseases later in life. The example set by adults' alcohol consumption is a very potent influence on youth, and therefore we are all part of the solution to limiting alcohol consumption to safer levels. A cultural change in our attitude to alcohol is required.

Sun protection

A second generation of Australians has now grown up with the 'Slip Slop Slap' summer campaigns which began in the 1980s. Since then, 'Seek' and 'Slide' have been added to the list to remind people to seek shade when the UV (ultraviolet light from the sun) is likely to cause sunburn, and to slide on sun glasses to protect their eyes. This is shown in Figure 3.5. Protecting against intense UV light from the sun will reduce the damage to the skin that causes skin cancer and premature ageing of the skin.

Slip on clothing that covers much of the skin. Loose clothing but with a tight weave is usually best. Some clothes have an ultraviolet protection factor (UPF). This should be a least 15 to offer good protection but improves to excellent at 50.

Slop on sunscreen to areas of the skin not covered by clothes. The sunscreen you use should be labelled at least SPF 30 (sun protection factor) although most these days will be SPF 50. (SPF 30 filters 96.7% UV while SPF 50 filters 98%.) It should be labelled broad spectrum which means it covers both the UVA and UVB (see below) and it should be labelled water resistant. Apply sunscreen 20 minutes before going out into the sun and reapply every 2 hours. Be generous with applying sunscreen, using at least ½ teaspoon to each arm, face, and neck, and one teaspoon for each leg as well as back and front.

Slap on a hat. Broad-brimmed hats give the best protection but bucket or legionnaire styles, particularly for children, protect face, ears, and neck.

Seek shade when the sun is intense in the middle of the day.

Slide on sunglasses to protect the eyes. In Australia and New Zealand, of categories 0 to 4, only 2, 3 and 4 give acceptable UV protection.

When you should protect against the sun depends on how intense it is, and that will vary by where you live. Weather reports now often include the UV Index for different times of the day in different locations. There is also a Sunsmart smart phone app available which will give you that information. If the index is 3 or above you need to take sun protection measures. If it is below 3 you can safely be exposed to the sun.

Sunlight consists of three different wavelengths. The long UVA rays penetrate deep into the skin and cause ageing, but also contribute to cancer by suppressing the immune system. The shorter length UVB are mainly responsible for sunburn of the skin. UVC is a shorter wavelength but is absorbed by the ozone layer in the upper atmosphere before it reaches us. UVB sunburn is not

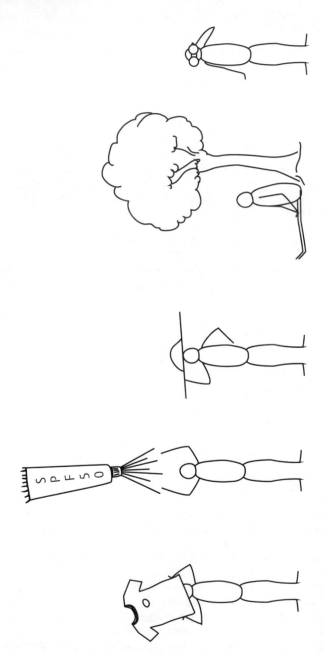

Figure 3.5 Slip, slop, slap, seek, slide.

only uncomfortable at the time, the damage can later on result in skin cancer. Cumulative damage predisposes to non-melanoma skin cancer while intermittent damage is more the pattern associated with the later development of melanoma. If you have been exposed to enough UVB to start to redden the skin then you have done sufficient damage to increase your risk of cancer.

You need some sun exposure because the action of UV in the skin is how vitamin D is produced. However, in the summer this amounts to only a few minutes to the equivalent of the face and arms each day. This should not be at a time when the sun is intense enough to cause sunburn (UV Index 3 and above) because that degree of damage is what can cause cancer and premature ageing of the skin later on. In the winter, where in many places the UV Index is mainly below 3, you need the equivalent of 3–4 hours of sun each week. For those people who cannot get even that degree of sun exposure, such as those who completely cover their skin for religious or cultural reasons or those who are too ill to be outside, vitamin D supplements should be considered.

Solariums are not safe ways of obtaining UV exposure. Some machines deliver UV more intensely than the sun and will damage the skin just like sun tanning will. The rate of skin cancer has been found to increase particularly in younger patients who use solariums regularly.

It is a myth that having a tan is healthy. The tanned look is a fashion often ascribed to Coco Chanel, the French fashion designer. So the story goes, in 1923 she accidentally became sunburned while on a yacht sailing to Cannes and when she appeared on the Riviera with a golden tan, this look became the fashion. Prior to that, the pale look was desirable. In some countries looking suntanned is still undesirable because it is associated with being a peasant and working out in the fields!

While we are talking about myths, there is an idea that getting a tan helps protect you from further sun damage. This is not true. The best protection a tan could achieve would be the equivalent to an SPF factor of 4! People with very dark skin have more protection than fair skinned people but they can still get skin cancer if the skin is damaged sufficiently by UV exposure. They also are prone to developing cancer on their less pigmented palms and soles.

Public education about sun protection is very important. Campaigns are run at the start of each summer and sun surveys are done to monitor people's behaviour. They show that sun protection has improved. Programmes in primary schools that require children to wear hats and sunscreen in the summer have been particularly successful. Unfortunately the group who most often get sunburnt in the summer are the late teens and young adults who give their major reason for a lack of sun protection as simply forgetting.

Sunscreen

Sunscreens should not be relied upon as the only form of sun protection since they are not 100% effective. They should be the final measure after covering up with clothing, hats, and sunglasses. Daily use of sunscreens in the summer has been linked with a decrease in the chances of developing skin cancer, but remember to reapply every 2 hours to maintain the effect.

It doesn't matter how much a sunscreen costs, if it is labelled as at least SPF 30 and broad spectrum it will give an adequate level of protection. The differences in sunscreens are usually to cater for personal preferences such as preference for a cream, lotion, or gel. Some people may develop allergic reactions to some sunscreens. If you do, try another product because they all have different preservatives in addition to the UV blocking chemicals and these other preservatives or perfumes may be responsible for the allergy or irritation. Sunscreens made for children's use are often freer of additional chemicals.

There has been some press given to formulations of sunscreens where the zinc or titanium UV blockers (zinc oxide or titanium dioxide) are refined down to nanoparticle size in order to make the sunscreens colourless. There are no studies that have found these small particles to be more harmful than the regular size.

Protecting your eyes

The best way of protecting your eyes is a broad-brimmed hat and close-fitting, wrap-around sunglasses. These protect against the light that comes from the front and the sides of your eyes. Protection is important because UV exposure can lead to skin cancers on the surface of the eye and eyelids. There are other problems such as cataracts and damage to the retina at the back of the eyes that will also be avoided. Protecting the eyes is particularly important in children, and adults with prolonged exposure to intense UV light as part of their jobs. If you spend a lot of time in your car, tinting the side windows can be helpful because although laminated windscreens block most of the UVB and can block UVA, the tempered glass of side windows often lets through more UVA.

If you think that getting skin cancer years later is a trivial matter, you need to know that over 2000 Australians die of skin cancer each year. The most lethal form of skin cancer is melanoma, often just a dark spot on the skin, and responsible for over 1500 deaths. There are over 12,000 of these diagnosed in Australia each year. There is the suggestion that climate change with depletion of the ozone layer will increase the number of skin cancers. Melanoma occurs decades after episodes of intense sun exposure causing sunburn rather than continuous exposure. Children who get sunburnt have almost twice the chance of developing melanoma later in life than those who don't. Melanomas are usually found in sun-exposed areas of the skin. The chance of it spreading beyond the skin is high and depends on how deep it is when discovered. That is why it is so important to get to know your skin and immediately report any change in size, shape, or colour of a spot on the skin. Certainly if you notice irritation or bleeding in a skin spot you should seek medical advice promptly. This should lead to a more prompt diagnosis than relying on annual skin checks which are better used for selected people at high risk. Once melanoma spreads it is still very difficult to cure despite some promising new targeted drugs. Solarium use increases the risk of melanoma particularly in young people and also is associated with more of the rarer melanomas found at the back of the eyes.

The two other most common skin cancers are called basal cell cancer (BCC) and squamous cell cancer (SCC). It is estimated that over 430,000 Australians present with these types of skin cancer each year. BCCs are twice as common as SCCs and both are more common in men than women. This is the type of skin cancer which is caused by more accumulated damage to the skin from regular exposure to high levels of UV light. Most probably the greater number of these skin cancers in men is largely due to more having jobs outside than women, with more continuous sun exposure. Although most of these can be cured by local treatment such as surgical removal, it is important to detect these as early as possible. Again, getting to know your skin and seeking advice as soon as you become aware of a change in one of the spots on your skin gives you the best chance of cure.

Some people are at higher risk of skin cancer than others. The prevention and early detection messages should be particularly heeded if you have fair skin, an increased number of unusual moles, a family history of melanoma in a close relative such as a mother/father or sister/brother, a previous skin cancer, or a condition which causes your immune system to be suppressed.

Once again, the measures to protect yourself from harmful sun exposure are simple, yet very effective in reducing your risk of skin cancer.

Safety at work

We spend a considerable proportion of our time at work and it is important to be aware of how we can prevent cancers that may occur because of workplace exposure. We have already discussed measures such as protecting against sun exposure in outdoor workers, having a smoke-free workplace, and making sure workers have access to healthy food. Other risks are due to exposures to specific chemicals as part of manufacturing or agricultural practices.

It is estimated that between 6% and 7% of cancers can be attributed to workplace exposures with much more exposure in men (nearly 11%) than women (around 2%) because of the differing nature of their work and workplaces. In Australia, over 50 different industries were identified as having the potential to expose workers to cancer-causing agents. The industries include the whole spectrum from agriculture and forestry through manufacturing to construction and retail. The most common cancers which occur because of these exposures are skin, lung, and bladder cancers.

The International Agency for Research on Cancer collects all the information available about chemicals that cause cancer and then ranks them as either certainly, probably, or possibly causing cancer. This is where we get a lot of our information about what exposures we need to protect against. Just to show how widespread the extent of this task is, there are 29 agents encountered in the workplace listed as certain to cause cancer and 28 listed as probable. Now it is important to say here that just because a chemical has the potential to cause cancer, whether it does or not depends on how much of it you are exposed to. With some chemicals you may need to be exposed to such a large amount that there will never be a problem. If you needed to be exposed to a swimming pool full and are only exposed to a thimble full then you won't get that type of cancer.

One of the best known occupational cancers is mesothelioma, a cancer of the outer lining of the lung and abdomen, caused by exposure to asbestos. Although asbestos is no longer produced or used as a building material in most Western countries, people may still be exposed when renovating old buildings. However, there are many other occupational exposures which increase the risk of cancer, including exposure to cadmium in the production of batteries which has been linked with lung cancer, exposure to aromatic amine dyes for dying fabrics which is linked to bladder cancer, and benzene exposure in the rubber industry linked to leukaemia. Hairdressers who are regularly exposed to hair dyes may be at higher risk of bladder cancers and lymphomas but this has not been established for individuals who dye their own hair. There are certain occupations such as house painters where there is a higher risk of cancer but no specific chemical has been identified. The occupations with the greatest numbers of workers exposed to agents which increase the cancer risk are the agriculture and forestry industries.

The best way of preventing cancer in these situations is to get rid of the agent causing the problem. That is not always practical or desirable so the next strategy is to protect yourself in workplaces with the appropriate clothing and eyewear or, where necessary, use special equipment like respirators.

Pesticides

Having mentioned agriculture it seems timely to discuss the link between pesticides and cancer. The problem here is that the word covers hundreds of chemicals and so it has been very difficult to establish whether pesticides cause cancer. There is no doubt that some of the chemicals are definite cancer-causing agents, so it will come down to the extent of exposure. The organo-chlorines and creosote are known to be cancer-causing chemicals while agents like DDT are tumour promoters.

Here, it makes sense to look at people exposed more regularly than the general population such as farmers, pesticide manufacturers, and applicators. There is a higher risk of leukaemia in these workers but it is a weak association and of course they are also likely to be exposed to many other cancer-causing chemicals like diesel exhausts and solvents.

At the other end of the scale, people are worried about whether pesticide residues on the fruit and vegetables that they eat increase their cancer risk. There is no evidence that eating fruit and vegetables increases cancer risk and as we have seen, the fruit and vegetable diet may decrease the risk. This lack of association is not a surprising result as the 'dose' of any residual pesticide would be extremely small.

There is one other note of caution about pesticides: there is a suggestion from research joining many studies together that parental exposure to pesticides may increase the risk of cancer in their children, particularly lymphomas and brain cancers.

Diesel engine exhaust

There is a definite link between exposure to diesel exhaust and cancer. The exhaust is a mixture of gases and small particles which are inhaled. However, the major risk is to workers exposed continually to diesel exhaust, such as professional drivers and some miners. This occupational exposure increases the risk of lung and bladder cancer.

Firefighters

Several large studies have suggested an overall increase in cancer incidence in firefighters. There has been some inconsistency in which cancers are associated with this occupation, but some studies have shown increased rates of prostate cancer and melanoma. Mesothelioma has also been reported to be increased, and that may be because of asbestos exposure in old buildings which catch fire. Protective clothing which protects the skin and respirators may reduce the exposure to cancer-causing agents for these workers.

Shift work

Shift work where sleep–wake cycles are being constantly disrupted is possibly responsible for developing cancer. The strongest association is with women working night duty and increasing their risk of breast cancer. The mechanism may be related to disruption of melatonin cycles, but more research is required.

Monitoring for future occupational cancers

As new materials become available for use in manufacturing, workers should be monitored for possible adverse effects of occupational exposure. One example is carbon nanotubes which can be used in the manufacturing of goods from tennis rackets to computer chips. The possibility that if inhaled they could set up similar chronic inflammatory effects as asbestos fibres has prompted the need to take precautions for those who would be exposed during manufacturing. Alternatively carbon nanotubes could become carriers to get drugs into cells and so may have the potential to be part of new cancer treatments. This simply shows that raising concerns about a product does not mean that it should not be developed, just that it requires care in protecting against possible adverse effects.

Population screening for cancer

There are currently three population screening programmes that have been found to be successful in preventing cancer and there are screening tests proposed in other cancers for specific high-risk groups within the population.

Cervical cancer screening

Cancer of the cervix is one of few cancers where a population screening test can either prevent cancer from developing, or if it has developed, detect it early when it is still possible to cure it. This is because it is possible to detect cells that have changed but are not yet cancer, so-called precancerous growth, and destroying them will prevent cancer occurring. These precancerous changes can develop over 10 years, so regular testing should detect them before cancer develops. Despite having a vaccine against human papilloma virus (HPV) which can prevent cancer of the cervix you still need to be screened, since the vaccine is only about 70% effective.

Currently a Pap test (named for Dr George Papanicolaou who developed it) involves inserting a speculum into the vagina and collecting cells from the cervix using the speculum and a brush. This screening test should commence for women between 18 and 20 years old or within 2–3 years of becoming sexually active and go to 70 years, repeating the test every 2–3 years. Since the introduction of the HPV vaccine there has been research that will see the Pap test replaced by testing for the presence of HPV genetic material (DNA) in the cells in the samples collected in a similar way. It is suggested that this HPV testing should occur every 5 years commencing at the age of 25 years. The benefits of cervical cancer screening can be demonstrated in Australia where the number of cases of cancer of the cervix and the number of deaths have halved since screening was introduced.

Breast cancer screening

Breast cancer is one of the few cancers which have a screening programme across the whole population. The target group, who are likely to have the most benefit, are women between the ages of 50 and 69. This is the age group in which three-quarters of breast cancers are diagnosed.

The screening test is a mammogram, which is an X-ray of the breast. In Australia, there was a reduction of just over one-fifth in the breast cancer death rate when the screening programme was introduced. There is, however, a debate over how much of that was due to breast screening and how much was due to improved treatments for breast cancer, and this debate continues worldwide as countries evaluate their programmes.

Screening of younger women aged 40–49 years can be offered, but the benefit is not as great compared to the risks. Technically the mammogram is less accurate because the breast tissue is denser and it is more difficult to identify a cancer. Women at high risk of developing breast cancer because of a strong family history may well be advised to begin screening in this age group. Other tests such as MRI (magnetic resonance imaging) are being verified to see if they are more accurate in younger women. Likewise, older women can be screened but they have less chance of benefit to offset the risks of screening, which include the cumulative exposure to radiation during multiple testing.

Bowel cancer screening

Bowel cancer is one of the three cancers for which population screening is offered. Kits for testing the bowel motions for blood are sent to people aged 50 years and over. A kit is shown in Figure 3.6. They are the faecal occult blood test (FOBT) which uses a chemical to detect the blood or the faecal immunochemical test (FIT) which uses antibodies to detect blood. When the programme is complete people will receive the test kits every 2 years until they are 74 years old. The kits consist of a small sampling probe and a tube in which the sample is sent off to the pathology laboratory for testing. Usually two or three separate bowel actions are tested.

This test works well as bowel cancer usually begins as non-cancerous polyps called adenomas that are small outgrowths of the bowel wall. This is shown in Figure 3.7. They grow slowly and those that become cancer often take at least 10 years for this to develop. Both cancers and polyps can cause bleeding (even if only microscopic amounts), and this is what the stool test detects.

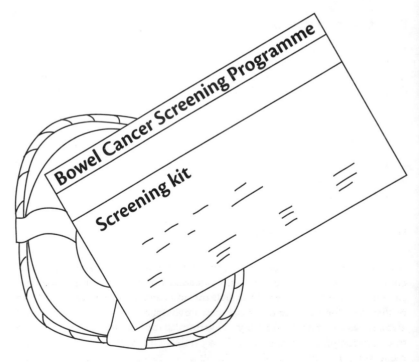

Figure 3.6 A bowel screening kit could be a life-saver.

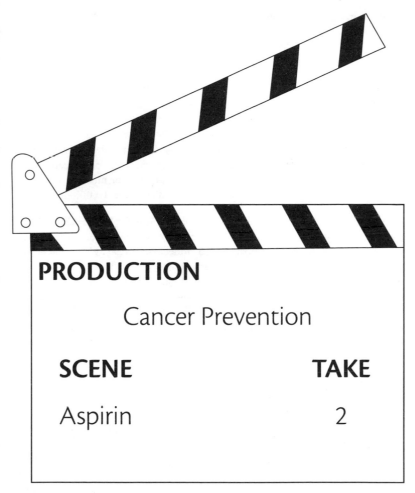

Figure 3.7 Could it be this simple

If tests are positive for blood then you are recommended to have a colonos-copy to have a look into the bowel. Under sedation, a flexible thin tube with camera and light are inserted through the anus and the large bowel wall can be inspected for polyps or cancers. Often a polyp that is not yet developed into a cancer can be removed during this procedure, thereby preventing cancer from developing. Cancers that are found are often very early in their develop-ment when they are more likely to be cured by surgery than those which are only found when symptoms develop.

About 1 in every 14 people tested will have a positive stool test. If a test is positive, at follow-up colonoscopy only 4.3% will have cancer and 48% will have polyps. The others will have benign conditions such as haemorrhoids as a cause for the bleeding.

It is estimated that screening will reduce deaths from bowel cancer by 30–40% and this is backed up by evidence of more bowel cancers being detected at early stages when they are more curable surgically, after bowel screening is introduced. There are no adverse effects of the bowel screening test except for the anxiety of having a positive test until the colonoscopy identifies the cause. A colonoscopy has rare adverse serious complications. The bowel can be perforated, which occurs in about 1 in 1000 colonoscopies or bleeding can occur in 1 in 1000 people. Deaths are rare but reported at 3–4 in 10,000 procedures.

There are other tests proposed to screen populations for bowel cancer. Some suggest going straight to colonoscopy but this would be expensive and there would be a large number of normal and unnecessary tests, given that selecting only those with positive FOBTs for colonoscopies focuses on the group more likely to have cancer and increases the likelihood of finding cancer at colonoscopy by up to 40 times. Flexible sigmoidoscopy has been suggested for screening, but it just examines the lower end of the bowel where 60% of cancers are found but cannot examine further than that. There are blood tests being developed to screen for bowel cancer but more trials are required to assess their accuracy.

Lung cancer screening

No one is suggesting that everyone should be screened for lung cancer, but the National Lung Screening Trial in the United States which showed a reduction in deaths from lung cancer of 20% by using three annual low-dose computerized tomography scans (LDCTs) to screen people at high risk of lung cancer, has opened the debate over whether such a high-risk group should be screened. The question most often raised after such research is 'Why wouldn't we want to start screening this group and improve the survival?' Well of course we do and if there if was no downside to screening and it was cost-effective we would probably immediately translate such research into practice. However, there are downsides to screening and it will help you see why there can be different interpretations of study results that determine whether a population screening test will be adopted.

Firstly, what is a high-risk group? The trial included people from age 55 to 74 who had a 30-year history of smoking a packet a day or who had quit 15 or fewer years ago. However, the United States Preventative Services Task Force extended this to from age 55 to 80 and recommended annual screening until the person had quit for 15 years. They also realized that occupation and other lung disease should be considered in assessing high risk. It is important to identify precisely which group will benefit the most.

What are the downsides to screening? Firstly you are being exposed to radiation. A LDCT scan delivers about ten times that of a chest X-ray and if you are having multiple scans or follow-up conventional scans it may be a cumulative dose that increases the risk of a second cancer.

The biggest problems with lung scans, however, are the very high percentage of nodules that are picked up that are not cancer (so-called false positive scans). In the US trial, over 96% of the scans were false positives on further investigation. Often nodules are simple scars from previous infections but the scan can't distinguish these from very early cancers. However, the positive scan triggers all the psychological distress caused by the possibility of having cancer. Even if the nodules are cancers, they may be so slow growing that they will never cause a problem in the patient's lifetime. This will occur with most screening programmes but has been estimated at over 18% of cancers found by LDCT. The problem is that these may trigger further investigations including biopsies, or worse, result in invasive treatments that essentially will not improve the survival from the lung cancer (so-called overtreatment).

The smallest issue for patients, but important for health regulators, is the cost. The ideal screening test is one which is cheap enough to roll out across a large population. CT scans are expensive compared to other screening tools such as FOBT kits as part of screening for bowel cancer. The other aspect of cost is the opportunity cost of what could be funded instead of these CTs to reduce the death rate from lung cancer. For example, the most cost-effective method for reducing mortality from lung cancer would be to put the money towards a tobacco control initiative.

So far there is only the one large trial reported, but there are others in progress which may influence decisions about whether to start screening high-risk groups for lung cancer. A Dutch/Belgium randomized lung screening trial is due for reporting in 2015 and a United Kingdom trial in 2016. These may add more information about the balance of efficacy and adverse effects. For example, the Dutch/Belgium trial has already shown that the number of false positive nodules can be reduced by analysing their volumes. Lung screening is a matter, for the moment, of 'watch this space'.

PSA testing

Of the other cancers suggested as candidates for screening, prostate cancer has caused the most debate. The PSA (prostate specific antigen) blood test, while specific for diseases of the prostate, is not specific for cancer which means it can trigger further tests such as biopsies unnecessarily. Moreover, while most experts now agree that there is not enough evidence of net benefit in doing a PSA blood test to suggest that the whole population be tested, what do you do for a man who requests testing? The problem is that for some men, being tested may save their lives but for most it will not, yet may ultimately result in a prostatectomy with serious side effects such as impotence and incontinence for a slow-growing prostate cancer that would never have been life-threatening.

What is suggested is that men who have no symptoms but who want reassurance should talk to their GPs about the pros and cons of having a PSA test. It they choose to have the test they should be in the age range 50–70 years and be tested every 2 years. (Men with risk factors such as a strong family history may choose to be tested earlier, say from 45 years.) Over the age of 70 there is very little research about the benefit of testing but certainly there will be no benefit unless the man is likely to live for at least 7 more years. When a PSA blood test is performed it has been found that the GP will gain no more useful information by adding a digital rectal examination (inserting a finger into the anus to feel the prostate) and so that is unnecessary at this time.

If the PSA test result is over 3.0 nanograms per millilitre then a biopsy will be recommended. If the biopsy shows a low-grade prostate cancer the man should be monitored regularly but not immediately offered an operation to remove the prostate because it may never cause a problem.

What we need is a better test that is more specific for prostate cancer and we need to be able to predict which cancers to treat. There is much ongoing research into this area, but for the moment, population screening is not recommended anywhere in the world.

Screening for other cancers

Screening for other cancers has been suggested but there are simply no tests that are proven to save lives if the whole population is tested. Even for skin cancer it is better for you to know what your skin normally looks like and report any change to spots on the skin as soon as they occur rather than wait for an annual skin check. The types of changes include spots that are growing, changing colour, or beginning to irritate or bleed.

For testicular cancer, rather than a regular routine of examining yourself, it is better to report swelling or discomfort as it is found. Similarly, reporting breast lumps as soon as an abnormality is noticed is encouraged over regular breast self-examination, although participating in the breast screening programme is encouraged as it will detect cancers earlier in their development than self-examination before they are big enough to be felt.

Vaccines to prevent cancer

The two vaccines in widespread use are not anticancer vaccines but vaccines against the viruses that predispose to cancer. They are the vaccine against HPV which is a necessary infection before cancer of the cervix develops and the vaccine against hepatitis B which predisposes to liver cancer. These vaccines do not treat cancer, they prevent cancer from developing. One day specific anticancer vaccines will also be developed.

HPV vaccine

Persistent infection with HPV causes almost all cancers of the cervix. It is a sexually transmitted infection. There are many subtypes of HPV but subtypes types 16, 18, and 45 are responsible for most cervical cancers and 16 and 18 cause about 70% of cases. Current vaccines work against either 2 or 4 subtypes but there are vaccines against nine subtypes being trialled, and these should increase the percentage of cancers likely to be prevented. HPV is also associated with cancers of the penis, vulva and vagina, and throat.

To prevent HPV infection, a vaccine is given to 11- to 13-year-old girls and currently involves three injections into the arm or leg muscle: an initial injection, the second at 1 or 2 months, and the third at 6 months. Australia also vaccinates boys from age 12 to 13. In excess of 6 million doses have been given and we now know that this is a very safe vaccine. Redness and pain at the injection site are the most commonly reported side effects. Allergy to the vaccine is as rare as with other vaccines and there are no other serious problems associated with its use.

Hepatitis B vaccine

Two of the major risk factors for developing cancer of the liver are having had an infection with hepatitis B virus (HBV) or hepatitis C virus (HVC). These viruses can be transmitted sexually or by blood transfusion or other exposure to infected blood. Hepatitis B can be passed from mother to infant. Hepatitis B will progress to a chronic (longstanding) infection in most infants but only in up to 5% of adults when their immune systems do not clear the virus. It is the chronic infection that damages the liver and can progress to liver cancer.

The best way of preventing HBV is to vaccinate newborns. A common schedule is to vaccinate at birth then give three more doses at 2 months, 4 months, then 6 or 12 months. If not vaccinated at birth, 10- to 13-year-olds who have not been vaccinated can receive two or three doses over 6 months. If you are an adult in a high-risk group you should consider vaccination. Individuals at high risk include people with close or sexual contact with individuals with hepatitis B or sex workers, migrants from countries where hepatitis B is common or Aboriginal and Torres Strait Islanders, haemodialysis and transplant recipients, intravenous drug users, and travellers to areas where hepatitis B is common.

The vaccine protects 95% of infants and adolescents but this figure declines after the age of 40 to 65–70%. The vaccine is used to prevent infection; it is not a therapy for those already infected.

Medication to prevent cancer

Most drugs that have been developed in the cancer field actually treat established cancer. However, we are seeing the emergence of drugs which may be used to prevent cancer from developing. This would be much simpler for some than embarking on major lifestyle changes. Two current examples are the use of tamoxifen or similar anti-breast cancer hormones for preventing breast cancer, and the emerging evidence of the impact of aspirin, particularly in preventing bowel cancer.

Tamoxifen

Tamoxifen is a drug commonly used to treat those breast cancers whose growth is stimulated by the female hormone oestrogen. However, it can be given to young women at high risk of developing breast cancer because of their strong family history, where it has been shown to be able to prevent the development of cancer if given daily over at least 5 years.

Aspirin

The common pain killer aspirin is often used in low doses to help prevent further events after heart attacks or strokes. When a large group of people who were taking aspirin for this purpose were evaluated for whether they later developed cancer, it was found that their incidence of bowel cancer was decreased. This is illustrated in Figure 3.7. People in the 50–65 years age group who had taken aspirin for at least 10 years cut the risk of bowel cancer by at least 35%. The chances of getting other cancers, such as oesophagus and stomach cancers, may also be reduced. A trial of aspirin among people who had inherited a high risk of bowel cancer showed similar impressive reductions in the incidence of cancer. More work needs to be done on which groups will benefit most, what is the best dosing and timing of the tablets, and where the balance lies between the benefits and side effects such as the increased risk of a gastric ulcer or bleeding. These issues need to be refined before this can be widely recommended, but such a simple cost-effective cancer prevention strategy is appealing.

Other risk factors

There are many other everyday exposures that are said to cause cancer but often evidence is lacking, or the studies that are performed reach opposite conclusions. Sometimes other illnesses associated with cancer such as depression can raise issues of whether they result from cancer or play some role in its cause. In the case of depression, more work is needed to determine whether anxiety or depression could cause some cancers.

New technologies such as mobile phones have come under scrutiny as to whether they can cause cancer. It has been suggested that brain tumours may be caused by the electromagnetic radiation from phones held close to the skull. So far, no definite link has been shown for ordinary usage up to 10 years but the jury is still out beyond that time. It is also not clear just how that lower-level radiation would actually trigger cancer. So, we may take precautions of limiting children's use of mobile phones and continuing to monitor large populations to correlate the extent of their usage with whether they develop cancer.

Similarly the low-level radiation in airport scanners has been questioned regarding their potential to cause cancer. Although it is unlikely, one has to ask why there would also not be a concern about the greater exposure of flying at high altitude for several hours?

There are numerous stories that are spread increasingly through social media about various potential causes of cancer, ranging from the use of underarm deodorants to drinking from plastic bottles after they have been left in the sun. Although there is no evidence to underpin such claims they seem to gain currency by repetition. Cancer Council Australia has a very good website, the iHeard site (http://iheard.com.au/), where people can ask about myths and rumours around cancer causes and it now has dozens of answers according to the latest scientific studies.

4

Risk factors and the prevention of specific cancers

Preventing common cancers

We have given general advice on preventing cancer, including details of healthy diets and how much exercise to do in Chapter 3, but you may want more details about specific cancers. After all, if you find that you have a family history of bowel cancer you will be keen to know what other risk factors you could modify to avoid developing that cancer. We have selected the top 20 common cancers worldwide, starting with the most common (including skin cancer which has high incidence but is not always included in lists because non-melanoma skin cancer statistics are not part of most cancer registries) to explore whether there is helpful information that you can use to prevent them.

Skin cancer

In Chapter 3 we covered the basics of preventing skin cancer by protecting your skin against the sun when it is intense enough to damage and burn your skin in the middle of the day, by covering up with clothing, hats, and sunglasses and applying sunscreen regularly. Avoiding tanning solariums was part of the advice because they often have the potential to deliver up to 12 times more intense UV radiation than the sun. Using solariums increases the chances of getting melanoma threefold and non-melanoma skin cancer by 1½ to 2½ times compared to the incidence in non-users. Getting to know your skin and seeking professional advice about any changes as soon as you find them is important for early detection.

In addition, some prescription medications may make your skin more sensitive to sunlight and extra precautions need to be taken. Examples include the tetracycline and sulphonamide antibiotics, anti-inflammatory drugs such as naproxen and ibuprofen, diuretics such as frusemide, the anti-diabetic sulpho-nylureas, as well as the chemotherapy drug 5-fluorouracil.

Other measures suggested for skin cancer prevention include tinting windows in cars and buildings. However, this would probably only be helpful for those exposed to direct sunlight through the windows for long periods, as laminated glass in windscreens is quite an effective filter of UVB radiation, without tinting.

Chemoprevention

Chemoprevention is a term for using drugs to prevent cancer. Several have been tried to prevent skin cancers. Beta-carotene tablets did not help and selenium may have even increased the risk of squamous cell skin cancers. Isotretinoin can have severe side effects but can prevent new skin cancers in a rare disease, retinitis pigmentosa, which results in a depigmented skin. Celecoxib slightly decreased the rate of non-melanoma skin cancer in patients with sun-damaged skin (solar keratoses) and although DFMO (alpha-difluoromethylornithine) stopped non-melanoma skin cancers recurring after the original diagnosis, these two drugs can also have serious side effects.

Treatment of solar keratoses

Actinic (or solar) keratoses are sun-damaged areas of skin which can become skin cancers. If treated early, skin cancers can be prevented. Isolated spots are usually frozen off with liquid nitrogen, but for more widespread dam-age, creams or gels are used. One method used is the topical application of a chemotherapy drug, 5-fluorouracil. Another, imiquimod cream, stimulates an immune response against the skin cancers. Ingenol mebutate is a gel which only requires 2 or 3 days of application. A further technique for these kera-toses and a superficial form of squamous cell cancer, Bowens disease, is to give a light sensitizer (like 5-aminolevulinic acid—5-ALA) to the affected area and activate it by shining blue or green light on it, which destroys the targeted area but leaves the normal skin alone.

Lung cancer

Steps to prevent lung cancer are vital because unfortunately, unless the cancer is found at a very early stage, very few people live to 5 years after diagnosis.

Tobacco

The major message for prevention is preferably never to smoke or at least to stop smoking, stop smoking, stop smoking. Ninety per cent of lung cancer in men is directly attributed to tobacco use and about 80% in women. It is never too late to stop smoking. Ten years after quitting you will have already reduced your chances of lung cancer by 50% compared to someone still smoking. It is important in the home or workplace to avoid second-hand smoke from others smoking around you as this also increases your risk of lung cancer. Heavy marijuana smoking has also been associated with a greater risk of developing lung cancer.

Radon

Radon is a gas which is found naturally in some soils and rocks. It is odourless and colourless but if your home is built in areas where this is present the exposure to it will increase your risk of lung cancer. You can have your house tested and there are methods for venting the gas which will make your home safer.

Occupational exposure

Exposure to asbestos is most often associated with the development of a rare cancer of the outer lining of the lungs, called mesothelioma, however it can also cause lung cancer. It is more likely to do so in people who smoke, and both blue and white asbestos have been associated with lung cancer. Although the exposure may be at work in asbestos mines, it may also have been used in old buildings or the brake linings of older cars or in ship building. There is a risk for the do-it-yourself home renovator who should learn to identify asbestos and have it removed by experts.

In any workplace such as mines or manufacturing plants where you could inhale cancer-causing chemicals you should be given the protection of face masks and adequate ventilation. You must also take care at home where the fumes from wood-burning stoves should be adequately ventilated.

Diet and exercise

Lung cancer is one of the cancers where a healthy diet which is low fat, high fibre, and with adequate fresh fruit and vegetables and whole grains may help reduce the risk. You should be cautioned, however, about taking supplements. For example, heavy smokers who took beta-carotene tablets actually increased their risk. Retinol and vitamin E supplements have also been questioned. Heavy drinking has also been associated with lung cancer. Along with diet, exercising regularly is also important in lung cancer prevention.

Breast cancer

Breast cancer is one of the cancers where there is an effective screening pro-gramme using mammograms for women at the highest risk, that is, between ages 50 and 69 years, although the 40 to 50-year-olds at high risk will also benefit. Between 5% and 10% of breast cancers are thought to be heredi-tary. The most common mutations are in the *BRCA1* and *BRCA2* genes, the former associated with up to an 80% lifetime risk of developing breast cancer. This means that high-risk members of the family of a patient who presents with one of the mutations can be tested. Women identified as carrying these mutations may opt to have their breasts and ovaries removed to reduce their chances of cancer but this decision should not be taken lightly. Removing the ovaries will create a premature menopause which can have a significant impact on a woman's quality of life.

Diet and exercise

Being overweight increases the chances of developing breast cancer after menopause, so a healthy diet with more fruit and vegetables and less fat and sugar, as well as regular exercise applies to breast cancer as well as many other cancers. Drinking alcohol also increases your risk of breast cancer.

Factors relating to female hormones

Women who have an early onset of menstrual cycles (before 12 years old) and late menopause (after the age of 55) have a slightly higher risk of breast cancer because of the longer exposure of the breasts to the female hormones oestrogen and progesterone. Having a baby before the age of 30 years can be protective and breastfeeding for the first year has also been found to be pro-tective. Hormone replacement therapy to alleviate symptoms of menopause has been found to increase the risk of breast cancer. Some women may have an increased risk of breast cancer while taking some oral contraceptives but this reverts to normal when they stop. Women with a mother, sister, or daugh-ter with breast cancer have twice the risk, where with two close relatives they have triple the risk compared to those with no family history. In these women, drugs that block oestrogens have been found to be protective. These include tamoxifen, raloxifene, and drugs known as aromatase inhibitors such as anas-trozole. These drugs may also be helpful for women who have had one hor-mone sensitive breast cancer and therefore have a three- to fourfold risk of a second breast cancer.

From the 1940s to the 1970s, the drug diethylstilboestrol (DES) was given to women to prevent miscarriages, but that was subsequently found to also increase their chance of developing breast cancer. There is emerging evidence of an increased risk of breast cancer for women doing night shifts but this needs more investigation and may be due to the levels of the hormone melatonin.

Tobacco

As with other cancers, the breast cancer risk is further increased in smokers.

Radiation

Exposure to high doses of radiation, even multiple CT scans, can increase the risk of developing breast cancer. Those who have had radiotherapy to the chest, for example, for Hodgkin lymphoma, have a higher chance of later contracting breast cancer.

Breast diseases

Some benign breast lumps that look as if they grow quickly are associated with an increased risk of breast cancer. Also, women who have denser breasts on mammograms are more at risk.

Bowel cancer

The good news with large bowel cancer is that 75% of this cancer could be prevented by screening and changing lifestyles. We emphasized the importance of large bowel screening in people aged 50 and over using a faecal occult blood test with follow-up of the positives by colonoscopy (see Chapter 3). Now we discuss how your risk can be further reduced. There is a group of bowel cancers that are inherited and a strong family history may mean screening at an earlier age. Patients with hereditary non-polyposis coli cancer (HNPCC) have been shown to reduce their risk by taking daily low-dose aspirin tablets for several years. More work is required to assess the risks and benefits of people at low or moderate risk of bowel cancer taking aspirin, since it can cause ulceration and bleeding. Those inheriting a condition with thousands of bowel polyps called familial polyposis coli should have their large bowels removed before the third decade to prevent the almost certain risk of developing bowel cancer. A polyp is shown in Figure 4.1. People with inflammatory bowel diseases are also more prone to developing bowel cancer.

Diet and exercise

With bowel cancer it is important to eat a diet relatively high in fruit and vegetables, and whole grains, with plenty of fibre, and to exercise regularly.

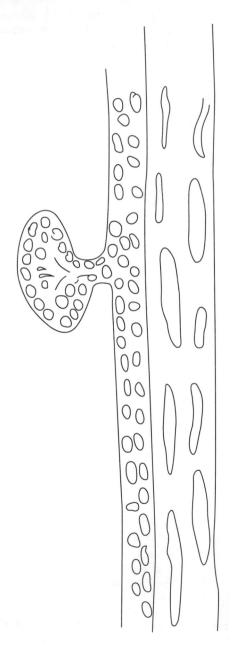

Figure 4.1 Polyps (adenomas) can precede bowel cancer by 10 years.

Consumption of red meat should be limited, especially processed meats like bacon, salami, and ham. Getting sufficient vitamin D and calcium seems important in reducing the risk of large bowel cancer and it has been suggested that folate is also important.

Alcohol and tobacco

Bowel cancer risk is increased both by alcohol and smoking. Fortunately these are modifiable risk factors.

Prostate cancer

Prostate cancer occurs predominantly in older men. A family history of prostate cancer increases your risk, particularly if your close relatives developed it before the age of 55 years. Prostate cancer is far more prevalent in Western cultures and this has been largely attributed to the Western meat-based diet.

Medication

A large trial of the 5-alpha-reductase inhibitor drugs finasteride or dutasteride in men with the benign swelling of the prostate called benign prostatic hypertrophy showed a reduction in prostate cancer of 25%, but those men who developed cancer were found to have more aggressive disease.

Maintain a healthy weight

Once again a balanced diet, watching your calorie intake, and reducing the fat from dairy and red meat is important, as well as eating cruciferous vegetables (cabbage, broccoli, cauliflower), tomatoes, and legumes. Fish with omega-3 fatty acids is often recommended although there is no proven guarantee of reducing your risk of prostate cancer by this dietary recommendation. It has been difficult to show a benefit from dietary supplements and high calcium intake has been suggested as increasing the risk. You can also reduce weight with regular exercise.

Stomach cancer

As an international problem, stomach cancer is the second leading cause of cancer deaths worldwide. It can occur in adults in their 20s, 30s, and 40s but most are over 55 years and most are men. The importance of prevention is highlighted by only 4% of patients surviving 4 years, often having presented late.

Risk factors include infection with *Helicobacter pylori* bacteria, inflammation of the stomach or polyps in the stomach, and pernicious anaemia which is due to a vitamin B_{12} deficiency. A family history of a close relative with stomach cancer or various genetic features such as having type A blood, inherited conditions associated with multiple polyps, and an inherited condition that affects multiple organs, the Li–Fraumeni syndrome, also increase the risk.

Diet

Dietary changes may reduce the risk of stomach cancer because of its association with diets poor in fruits and vegetables, particularly citrus fruits with vitamin C and vegetables with beta-carotene. The risk is also high if the diet contains a lot of foods preserved by salting or smoking. High-salt diets may also increase the risk in their own right. Being overweight and not getting enough exercise can impact on stomach cancer as well as many other cancers.

Environmental

Exposure to radiation can result in stomach cancer. Certain industries like the rubber, metal, and coal industries, or where you are exposed to asbestos, have higher rates of stomach cancer and therefore workers need to be protected against these workplace exposures.

Smoking

Stomach cancer is one of the smoking-related cancers and the risk will decrease if you stop smoking or have never smoked. It is probable, as with the head and neck cancers, that alcohol consumption with smoking also plays a role.

Aspirin

The use of aspirin is particularly associated with lowering the risk of bowel cancer but is also associated with a lower risk of stomach cancer. It is not yet clear whether aspirin should be taken specifically for this purpose because of the balance of the benefits with adverse effects, particularly bleeding.

Liver cancer

Liver cancer often develops in a liver that has been damaged. It may have become scarred (cirrhotic) by chronic alcohol use or infected with hepatitis B or C. It most often occurs in men over 60 years. Screening for liver cancer is not recommended for everyone except if you are in a high-risk group such as being Asian or African from regions where hepatitis B is widespread and having the infection or a family history of liver cancer, or other individuals with cirrhosis. Inherited diseases like haemochromatosis (iron overload of the liver) also predispose to liver cancer.

Alcohol and tobacco

Limiting alcohol reduces the risk of cirrhosis which can result in liver cancer. If you do drink alcohol, limiting this to two standard drinks a day should be safe. Liver cancer is yet another cancer where the risk is increased in smokers.

Hepatitis B and C

About 80% of primary liver cancers arise after viral hepatitis. A vaccine is available for hepatitis B which offers 90% protection of children and adults to prevent the infection and the subsequent risk of liver cancer. There is no vaccine for hepatitis C but your risk of contracting the infection can be reduced. It is sexually transmitted so knowing whether a partner is infected or practising safe sex with condoms will reduce the risk of transmission. It can also be transmitted by exposure to infected blood through sharing needles for drug use, or tattooing. Blood supplies for transfusion are now screened to prevent transmission by that route. People who have already been infected with hepatitis B or C can be offered medication to help reduce the liver damage.

Maintain a healthy weight

To prevent the possibility of developing non-alcoholic fatty liver disease, maintain a healthy weight by eating a diet which is low in fat and salt and high in fruit and vegetables and get plenty of exercise. Damaging the liver in this way is more common if you also have type 2 diabetes, high cholesterol, and high blood pressure so all of these should be controlled.

Chemical exposures

Depending on how grain is stored in developing countries it may become contaminated with aflatoxin, a mould which can cause liver cancer. Exposure to arsenic through drinking water can also be problematic. Use of anabolic steroids (in body building, for example) has been associated with an increased risk of liver cancer.

Cervical cancer

Cancer of the cervix is one of the great success stories in terms of screening and prevention. The Pap test screening programme has been highly effective where implemented, to identify pre-invasive cancers and early cancers when they can be curatively treated. In addition, there is now a vaccine against the human papilloma virus (HPV) which infects the cervix before cervical cancer can develop. This will reduce that infection by 70%. Unfortunately lower socioeconomic status and some ethnic groups are associated with a high rate of cervical cancer because they are less likely to participate in screening or vaccination.

HPV infection

HPV can be spread through sexual intercourse or skin-to-skin contact. Using condoms is estimated to reduce the rate of infection by 70% and reducing the number of sexual partners and increasing the age at which you first have sex are ways of reducing the risk of infection. Many infections can be cleared but some persist and start changing the cells in the cervix towards becoming cancerous.

Infection with the human immunodeficiency virus (HIV), the virus that causes AIDS, also puts women at higher risk of HPV infection. For that matter, any immunosuppression such as medication to suppress the immune response with organ transplants or autoimmune diseases will likewise increase the chances of HPV infection. Women who have had chlamydia infections are also at greater risk of also having HPV infection.

Smoking

It is estimated that smoking doubles the risk of women getting cancer of the cervix as compared to non-smokers. Tobacco products are absorbed and can damage the nuclear material in the cervical cells as well as suppress the immune system's ability to fight HPV.

Diet

Once again, a diet low in fruit and vegetables is associated with a greater risk of cancer of the cervix. Obesity is also a risk for adenocarcinoma of the cervix.

Hormonal factors

The prolonged use of oral contraceptives in one study doubled the risk of cancer of the cervix if taken for 5 years, but this risk returned to normal 10 years after stopping. Of interest, if a woman has ever used an intrauterine contraceptive device (IUD) the risk of cancer of the cervix is reduced. Having three or more pregnancies seems to increase the risk of cervical cancer either as a marker of increased exposure to HPV or an immune suppressant effect, allowing the infection. Women who are younger than 17 years with their first pregnancy have a greater risk of developing cancer of the cervix as compared to those whose first full-term pregnancy is not until they reach 25 years old. Unfortunately, 1 in 1000 of the daughters of women who were treated with DES to try to maintain 'at-risk' pregnancies, develop clear cell cancers of the vagina and cervix. This practice stopped in the 1970s.

Oesophageal cancer

Cancer of the oesophagus is most common in men over 50 years.

Alcohol and tobacco

As for the other cancers in the head and neck regions avoiding alcohol and tobacco reduces the risk of oesophageal cancer, which is higher if they are used together.

Obesity

Being obese is a risk factor for cancer of the oesophagus and again, a healthy diet is one rich in fruit and vegetables, particularly those that are green and yellow, and cruciferous vegetables. Some have linked cancer of the oesophagus with deficiencies of beta-carotene, vitamin E, selenium, and iron.

Barrett's oesophagus and reflux

Reflux of acid from the stomach can damage the lining of the lower oesophagus and predispose to cancer. Chronic changes in this lining are known as Barrett's oesophagus. Some studies suggest that aspirin or even statins such as rosuvastatin, used for lowering cholesterol, may reduce the risk of developing oesophageal cancer from Barrett's oesophagus. Reflux can be treated with proton pump inhibitor drugs such as omeprazole, or even corrected surgically.

Other conditions

Cancer of the oesophagus is more common in people who have other head and neck cancers, or lung cancer, or have HPV infection. Likewise there is an association with a condition called achalasia where the valve at the end of the oesophagus does not open properly, and a rare inherited condition called tylosis where people have overgrowth of skin on the palms and soles. People with oesophageal webs are more prone to developing cancer. The unfortunate accident of ingesting cleaning fluids with lye (also known as sodium hydroxide) also causes damage which can become cancer.

Bladder cancer

It is difficult to prevent bladder cancer, which occurs in men four times more commonly than women and increases with age, rarely appearing before 40 years, but there are a few things that may reduce your risk. If you have had bladder cancer you should be followed up closely because it has the highest rate of returning after the first cancer, at 50–80%.

Smoking

There is a strong link between smoking and bladder cancer so stopping smoking reduces your risk.

Diet

The usual healthy dietary advice applies but with bladder cancer it is also important not to become dehydrated as fluids dilute any cancer-causing chemicals that may reach the bladder.

Industrial chemicals

There is a range of industrial chemicals including benzenes and arylamines that people working with dyes, such as hairdressers, or working in rubber, printing, paint, leather, plastics, textile, or dry cleaning plants are exposed to and truck drivers can be exposed to diesel exhaust. They should all be protected against these exposures. Exposure to arsenic in the water supply is also a risk factor for bladder cancer.

Other conditions

Infections with tropical parasites should be avoided as they can be associated with bladder cancer. It is suggested that chronic bladder infections and kidney stones may predispose to bladder cancer, but although this is not certain, these conditions should always be treated promptly. Cyclophosphamide is an anticancer drug that has a side effect of raising the risk of bladder cancer because of a breakdown product in the urine. People who have had kidney transplants are more prone to bladder cancer as well.

Lymphoma

The majority of lymphomas (cancer of the lymph glands) can't be prevented because the exact cause is unknown. Lymphomas have two age peaks, 15–40 years old and 55 years or older. They are more common in men and there can be a family history. There may be general factors such as obesity linked to poor diet and lack of exercise which is associated with the development of a lymphoma.

Infections

HIV is associated with the development of lymphoma. Again, any cause of a weak immune system such as an autoimmune disease can also be linked to the development of lymphoma as can the use of immunosuppressant drugs to treat patients who have had organ transplants. The human T-cell lymphoma/leukaemia virus HTLV-1 which is most common in countries like Japan and the Caribbean causes a skin-related lymphoma. The Epstein–Barr virus which causes glandular fever can also predispose to lymphomas but this cannot really be prevented.

The infection caused by the bacteria *Helicobacter pylori* affects the wall of the stomach and can cause ulceration and bleeding of the stomach lining, but is also associated with lymphoma. It can be treated with antibiotics and antacids but often is not detected because it may not cause symptoms, and more research is needed to determine if eradicating this does reduce the development of lymphoma.

Environmental chemicals

There are farming chemicals or fertilizers that have been associated with lymphoma as have industrial chemicals in the manufacture of rubber and glues. Asbestos and arsenic exposure increase the risk of lymphoma as does exposure to Agent Orange.

Cancer treatments

It is an unkind fact that using chemotherapy or radiotherapy to treat cancer can disrupt the genetic material to result in second cancers many years later. This is not common but when it does happen most patients have survived the first cancer only to develop the second, which is commonly a leukaemia or lymphoma.

Leukaemia

There are many types of leukaemia, which is a cancer of the white blood cells. Essentially there is acute leukaemia which is a sudden-onset disease and chronic leukaemia which is more of a prolonged illness. There are two main white blood cell types affected: either the myeloid cells or lymphocytes. In adults, acute myeloid leukaemia is more common and has a better outcome than acute lymphocytic leukaemia, whilst in children, acute lymphoblastic leukaemia is the more common and has a very high cure rate. For the purposes of prevention, most of what is known applies to acute leukaemias.

Inherited factors

Leukaemia can run in families. In children, having a brother or sister with leukaemia increases their risk of being diagnosed with leukaemia; if they are a twin, it is a high one in five chance. There are congenital disorders such as Down syndrome which are associated with a high chance of acute childhood leukaemias and there are also inherited immune system diseases which will predispose to leukaemia.

Environmental factors

High-dose radiation is linked with developing leukaemia some 6–8 years after exposure as documented in survivors of the atomic bomb over Nagasaki. Radiation exposure of the fetus may also later predispose to leukaemia. There are chemicals, especially benzene, where workers have been reported as developing leukaemia after several years and as with lymphomas, leukaemias are the most common second cancers following some types of cytotoxic anticancer chemotherapy. Smoking tobacco is a risk factor for developing acute myeloid leukaemia. The HTLV1 virus is associated with an uncommon T-cell leukaemia. Other possible modifiable causes such as pesticides or living in proximity to power lines are still being investigated.

Pancreatic cancer

Fortunately, cancer of the pancreas is less common than some of the other cancers. The position of the pancreas is shown in Figure 4.2. It responds poorly to treatment with only a 16% 5-year survival which falls to 2% if it has spread beyond the pancreas. Most patients are older than 55 years. Between 5% and 15% have a family history or they have other genetic mutations including in the *BRCA2* gene, which is more associated with breast and ovarian cancers. Many of the risk factors are in common with other cancers.

Obesity

Obesity is associated with pancreatic cancer. Recommendations are the same as for other cancers—more exercise and a diet containing fresh fruit and vegetables, with a controlled amount of fat and modest servings of lean meat.

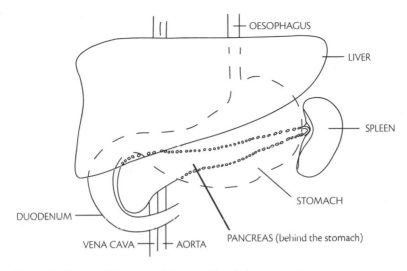

Figure 4.2 Organs of the upper abdomen. Where's the pancreas?

A possible relationship to more specific elements like alcohol and coffee are still to be absolutely proven.

Smoking

Smoking is a risk factor in around 20–30% of pancreatic cancers and quitting decreases the risk over time.

Environment

Various pesticides and industrial chemicals have been generally implicated in the development of pancreatic cancer. There may be a role for aspirin in reducing the risk, but further study is required.

Kidney cancer

Kidney cancer typically occurs between the ages of 50 and 70 years, and men are two to three times more likely to be diagnosed than women. People with a family history of the disease in parents, brothers or sisters, or children are at greater risk particularly if there are multiple relatives who were diagnosed before the age of 50 and had more than one cancer in the same or both kidneys. Inherited cancers account for only about 5% of kidney cancers and there are a group of rare genetic diseases with exotic names like von Hippel–Lindau syndrome which are associated with developing kidney cancer. In general, the causes of kidney cancer are not well understood and much of the prevention advice is general.

Tobacco and alcohol

Smoking doubles the risk of developing kidney cancer and is said to be responsible for 30% of cases in men and 25% in women, so quitting is clearly a way to reduce your risk. For some reason, consuming moderate amounts of alcohol in studies decreases the risk of kidney cancer but this is not a reason to start drinking and does not suggest drinking more than the general recommendation of a maximum of two standard drinks each day.

Obesity

Obesity is a risk factor, so a healthy diet with exercise is important in reducing the risk of kidney cancer, as it is for many other cancers.

High blood pressure

Men with high blood pressure are more likely to develop kidney cancer so blood pressure should be controlled.

Medications

There were painkillers sold over the counter which contained phenacetin which are now banned because of their link with kidney cancer, but care should also be exercised using other pain killers such as aspirin, paracetamol, as well as some diuretics.

Industrial exposures

The metal cadmium has been linked to kidney cancer. Exposure would occur in people working with batteries, paints, or welding. The risk is greater in workers who also smoke tobacco. Other exposures increasing the risk of kidney cancer include asbestos, coke used for steel making, benzene and other organic solvents, and herbicides. Workers should be protected from exposure to these cancer-causing agents.

Long-term dialysis

Patients on long-term dialysis can develop cancerous cysts in their kidneys which require removal.

Endometrial cancer

The risk of endometrial cancer (cancer of the lining of the uterus or womb), can be modified by avoiding some risks and adopting some protective practices. There are some factors beyond your control and these are the associations with inherited disorders, particularly HNPCC, and polycystic ovary syndrome. One study showed that doing hysterectomies in HNPCC reduces the risk of these women developing endometrial cancer. Without this intervention 30% developed endometrial cancer within 7 years.

Hormones

Exposure to the female hormone oestrogen increases the risk of endometrial cancer. In the natural cycle of events those women who have an early onset of menstruation and late menopause, which exposes them to oestrogens for longer, are at increased risk. Also at risk are those women who never have a baby as compared to those who do, who have more favourable hormone levels associated with pregnancy. Multiple pregnancies may be more protective as may breastfeeding for at least 12 months. If the hormone replacement therapy used for women after the menopause is only oestrogen, the risk of endometrial cancer is increased. If oestrogen is combined with progestin, the risk of endometrial cancer is not increased but that of breast cancer is, so you need to consult a professional about how to balance the risks and benefits in your particular situation. Using oral contraceptives for at least 1 year can also reduce the risk of endometrial cancer.

Tamoxifen, which blocks the effects of oestrogen on the breast, actually acts like oestrogen on the endometrium and if used for more than 2 years increases the risk of endometrial cancer. To prevent this, regular ultrasounds of the uterus should be done to see if the endometrium is growing thicker and if removed at that stage, this prevents cancer developing.

Smoking tobacco

Quitting tobacco use will reduce your risk of endometrial cancer.

Obesity

Being overweight is linked to endometrial cancer so diet and exercise are very important in modifying your risk of developing this cancer. Diets should certainly be low in fats.

Head and neck cancer

Head and neck cancer is a term used to refer to a number of different cancers spanning the lips to the throat, because they all have the same type of cell lining them. They are two to three times more common in men than women and usually develop in people over 40 years of age. The major risk factors are tobacco use and alcohol consumption.

Smoking tobacco and drinking alcohol

Eighty-five per cent of head and neck cancers are associated with tobacco use. Exposure to second-hand smoke also increases the risk. Smokers have up to a 35 times higher chance of developing head and neck cancer than non-smokers. However, it is never too late to quit smoking since even people with head and neck cancer who quit reduce their chance of getting a second cancer by up to 60%.

Alcohol is also a risk factor, increasing the risk two- to fivefold, but if combined with tobacco use the risk can be up to 100 times that of non-smokers and non-drinkers. Smokers of marijuana may also be at higher risk.

Betel nut

In countries like India and throughout South East Asia where betel nut chewing is common, there is an increased risk of cancers of the lining of the mouth. Betel nut has been implicated as causing these head and neck cancers even when it is not combined with tobacco. Chewing tobacco has also been associated with mouth cancer.

Sun exposure

The lips can be very sensitive to sun exposure and the risk of cancer, and require the same preventative measures that apply to skin cancer to avoid damaging the lips when the sun is intense. At least an SPF 30+ sun protection product should be used.

Occupational exposures

There are many occupational and environmental exposures that increase your risk of head and neck cancer. They range from asbestos exposure, paint fumes, and industrial chemicals like benzenes to wood dust. Your workplace should be adequately ventilated and you should be protected by using a mask or ventilator as necessary. Radiation exposure can also predispose to cancer in the head and neck region but is a higher risk to the glands, particularly the thyroid gland.

Viruses

Although better known for causing cancer of the cervix, the human papilloma virus (HPV) is associated with cancer of the nasopharynx (the part of the throat adjacent to the nose). This is a sexually transmitted virus and although safe sex is important, the use of condoms will not always prevent infection, and having multiple partners is a higher risk factor. Vaccination of boys as well as girls will help reduce the occurrence of this type of head and neck cancer. The other virus associated with nasopharyngeal cancer is the Epstein–Barr virus most associated with glandular fever. HIV causes AIDS (human immunodeficiency syndrome) and is associated with a high incidence of head and neck cancer. This is the case with any cause of immune deficiency. The herpes simplex virus (HSV) had been linked to mouth cancers, but the links with head and neck cancer are not as strong as the viruses mentioned earlier.

Dental hygiene

Head and neck cancer has been linked to poor gum and dental hygiene and at least annual dental checks are worthwhile. If you wear dentures it is important that they fit well. Cancer-causing chemicals from tobacco and alcohol could become trapped by ill-fitting dentures.

There are precancerous changes which may be detected by the dentist. Changes that appear as white plaques (leucoplakia) may not proceed to cancer and can resolve if exposure to tobacco and alcohol ceases.

Poor nutrition

A diet that is low in vitamins such as vitamin A and B is linked to an increased risk of head and neck cancer. Essentially this is a diet poor in fresh fruit and vegetables. Adding low fat, high fibre, and whole grains to a wide selection of fruit and vegetables provides the ideal diet to prevent many conditions.

Reflux

Reflux of acid up into the throat from the stomach is often experienced as indigestion or chest pain. It has also been linked to developing cancer in the throat, but usually can be easily treated.

Family history

If you have a history of head and neck cancer in close relatives this increases your risk, more so with very close relatives. The increased risk is even greater if you also smoke. Head and neck cancers are being investigated for what gene changes they may have, and there are some mutations that are commonly found, which raises the future possibility of targeting treatments against them.

Thyroid cancer

Thyroid cancer is typically diagnosed between 22 and 55 years and is three times as common in women as men. One type, papillary cancer, is typically found in women of childbearing age. There is an inherited thyroid cancer, medullary cancer of the thyroid, where if your parent has the responsible mutated gene you have a 50% chance of developing that cancer. A precautionary thyroidectomy may be advised. Other inherited conditions like hereditary polyposis includes thyroid cancer in the multiple organs affected.

Radiation

Exposure to radiation, particularly X-rays during childhood, predisposes to thyroid cancer later in life. In adults, exposure to radiation from, say, nuclear power plants, can cause thyroid cancer. This can be partly alleviated by taking iodine which floods the thyroid so that it can't take up the radioactive iodine.

Iodine deficiency

In many Western countries iodine is added to salt but iodine deficiency can be a problem in developing nations with inland populations where little fish or shellfish is eaten and this deficiency can predispose to thyroid cancer. Other iodine-containing foods include dairy, eggs, parsley, bananas, kelp, and vegetables like potatoes, radishes, and onions.

Brain cancer

There is much to be discovered about the causes of brain tumours and therefore little to be advised about prevention. They increase in frequency with age but there are specific types that occur in children and young adults. While they may not be directly inherited they are associated with some rare inherited conditions including Li–Fraumeni syndrome, von Hippel–Lindau disease, neurofibromatosis, and tuberous sclerosis.

Radiation

Children who receive high levels of radiation are more prone to brain tumours later in life.

Immune disorders

People who have AIDS are more likely to develop brain tumours as are those with lymphomas which are accompanied by suppression of the immune system.

Ovarian cancer

There are three main types of ovarian cancer depending on whether the cancer arises from the outer covering (epithelial type), the hormone-producing cells (stromal type), or the egg-producing cells (germ cell type). Most of this section refers to the 90% that are epithelial. The risk of a woman developing ovarian cancer increases with age, with 68% older than 55 years. Having a mother, daughter, or sister with ovarian cancer triples your risk of developing it. Around 10–15% of ovarian cancers occur because of inherited genetic mutations such as in the *BRCA1* and *BRCA2* genes, in common with breast cancer. Having breast cancer without these mutations also seems associated with an increased risk of ovarian cancer. There are other inherited conditions such as HNPCC which increase the risk of ovarian cancer along with other cancers including bowel and brain.

Hormonal factors

Anything that can prevent a woman ovulating, where an egg is released from the surface of the ovary which then has to be repaired by cells dividing, will reduce the chances of developing ovarian cancer. Women with early-onset menstruation and late menopause are at increased risk, as are those who have never had children or had their first child after they were 30 years old, have infertility, or have never used birth control tablets. Lesbian women seem at greater risk probably because of the greater representation of the mentioned earlier risk factors. Female transsexuals receiving hormones are at greater risk. Women who take oestrogen-only hormone replacement therapy after menopause are also at increased risk of ovarian cancer.

Therefore, having a child before the age of 30, breastfeeding, and taking birth control tablets reduce the risk. Taking birth control tablets for 3 years reduces the risk by 30–50%, particularly reducing the risk in people with *BRCA* mutations. However, the risk of breast cancer may increase, so you should seek advice which includes all of your risk factors.

Obesity

Once again obesity is a risk factor that brings in the need for a healthy diet and regular exercise. Women who are obese in early adulthood have a 50% greater chance of developing ovarian cancer than those who are not.

Hysterectomy

Women who have had a hysterectomy or have had their tubes tied to prevent conception have a reduced risk of developing ovarian cancer. If a hysterectomy is required on a postmenopausal woman, sometimes the tubes and ovaries are removed to reduce the risk of cancer.

Salpingo-oophorectomy

Some women with a strong family history or who find that they carry a *BRCA* mutation choose to have their tubes and ovaries removed to prevent ovarian cancer and fallopian tube cancer. If a premenopausal woman has her ovaries removed, the risk of ovarian cancer is reduced by 85–90% and the risk of breast cancer also reduces by 50%.

Gallbladder cancer

Gallbladder cancer is twice as frequent in women as men, as is developing gallstones. Most people are in their 70s before the disease develops. There can be a family history but both this and the cancer are rare.

Gallstones

Gallstones are a risk factor as they can cause inflammation, yet gallstones are so common and gallbladder cancer so rare that removing the gallbladder is usually not recommended just for the presence of stones. A porcelain gallbladder, where the wall is covered with calcium deposits, can be associated with long-term inflammation caused by gallstones and leads to a higher risk of gallbladder cancer which is also related to chronic inflammation.

Weight

Being overweight is a risk factor for both gallstones and gallbladder cancer and so a healthy diet and regular exercise are important.

Bile duct abnormalities

Cysts in the bile ducts (choledochal cysts) where the lining can develop cancer are a risk factor for gallbladder cancer. Other abnormalities of the ducts which allow backflow of pancreatic juices up the ducts also predispose to gallbladder cancer. Polyps in the gallbladder itself, particularly those over 1 centimetre in diameter can become cancerous. Primary sclerosing cholangitis where the bile ducts become inflamed and scarred, often in association with the inflammatory bowel disease ulcerative colitis, is also associated with an increased cancer risk.

Infections

People who become chronically infected with *Salmonella*, the bacterium that causes typhoid, or are typhoid carriers have a high risk of gallbladder cancer, probably because of the inflammation caused. Preventing infection with liver flukes by being careful with shellfish and eating only cooked fish in environments where this infection could be in waterways reduces the cancer risk. Preventing hepatitis as we outlined for liver cancer is also important in reducing the risk of gallbladder cancer.

5

Research into cancer risk

The spectrum of research

Most of what we currently know about the causes of cancer—which cancers have tests that are suitable and accurate enough for population screening, and how to treat cancer—have come from the evidence gathered by ongoing research. There are many different research methods. Laboratory research often studies isolated cells and what makes them grow, or uses model systems of cancers to investigate what influences their development. For new treatments, clinical trials are performed, ultimately comparing the old treatment with the proposed new treatment to see which is better in groups of patients who have the cancer being studied. Patients may also be interviewed to study their experience of cancer so that we may determine how best to improve that experience. To find what causes cancer, however, large populations need to be studied.

Why do we need to do research? Why aren't personal experiences of patients with cancer who recount exposures to various agents in our environment sufficient to inform us? Surely with a new treatment, if the outcome of the treatment in a particular cancer is well known, it will be obvious when a new treatment performs better than the old one did? What we need to discuss first is why we can't simply rely on individual experiences or comparing old with new treatments over time.

Let's start with the causes of cancer. One of us had a patient with breast cancer who found a breast lump and was sure that it developed after she had been hit in the breast by a tennis ball during a game a few weeks before. She believed that this triggered her cancer.

We know that this is not the case. Firstly, it takes up to a couple of years for a breast cancer to start from a single cancerous cell and grow big enough to feel, and so the timing of the trauma and the development of the cancer do not match. Secondly, research into the causes of breast cancer over large populations of people has not shown that trauma triggers breast cancers. People like to search for a reason for them developing cancer. In the case mentioned earlier, the injury to the breast probably caused the women to feel her breast and so she discovered the cancer early, before she developed more obvious signs, but that does not mean that the event preceding her finding the breast cancer caused it.

It is worth knowing that cancer rarely has a single cause. It often takes multiple 'hits' on the genetic material in the centre of the cell before a cancer is triggered. You may be born with some of the abnormalities or mutations in the genes and acquire others from the environment over many years (e.g. by smoking or what you eat, or exposure to cancer-causing chemicals). Unless you have one of the very strong risk factors like smoking or asbestos exposure it may be very difficult for you to isolate any particular single cause.

Moving to the reason that we need to do clinical trials instead of just comparing the outcomes of a new treatment with how the old treatment has performed over the years, we can illustrate this with the following example. It starts with what has become known as the Will Rogers phenomenon. Will Rogers was an American comedian who was attributed to making the unkind observation 'When the Okies left Oklahoma and moved to California, they raised the average intelligence level in both states.' In the one sentence he manages to insult those people who in his view were silly enough to migrate from Oklahoma as being of low IQ, but still brighter than anyone who actually lived in California before the migration. It is a clever comedy line, but what has this got to do with cancer research?

Let's take the case of locally advanced stage 3 sarcoma (a cancer of supporting tissue like muscle and bones) and stage 4 sarcoma that has spread to the lungs. Over the decades the survival of patients with both stages has improved. What a triumph for the benefit of the new treatments for sarcoma you may be tempted to believe. But no, there was no improvement in the treatment of sarcoma.

The reason for the apparent improvement in the survival from both stages 3 and 4 sarcoma was the introduction of the CT scan! Prior to the CT scan, the imaging of the lungs was done by chest X-ray which could only detect relatively large secondary cancers. When the CT scanner was introduced, very much smaller spots in the lungs could be seen. And so, those cancers which were originally counted with stage 3 but were actually stage 4 (you just could not see the secondaries on chest X-ray) suddenly were taken out of the stage 3 group after the CT scan. With the 'worst' of the stage 3 sarcomas gone, the survival improved. The stage 4 group now included patients with very small early lung secondaries and as a result, the survival of stage 4 sarcomas improved as well.

The lesson to be learned here is that if you want to test whether a treatment is responsible for improving the survival of a cancer you must compare the old and the new treatments under exactly the same conditions, where the only difference between the patients selected for each treatment group is the treatment itself. We will start with how trials of new cancer treatments are conducted as a background to how trials are done to discover what causes cancer.

Clinical trials of new treatments

Let's take the example of new anticancer drugs. They come from many different sources. Some are found by testing natural products against cancers in the laboratory. Some are made to hit genetic targets on cells that are known to promote cancer growth and some are just found by chance. When a drug has shown activity in laboratory systems and is ready to go into clinical trials, the first trial in humans, a so-called phase one study, is designed to find the maximum tolerated dose according to what side effects it has. Starting at a very low dose guided by the dosing in small animals, the dose is gradually escalated in groups of three patients until side effects limit the dose that can be given. A dose below that is identified as the dose for the phase two trials of efficacy.

In the efficacy trials, a group of patients with a particular tumour type is tested to determine whether the cancer responds to the drug by shrinking. It usually requires about 40–50 patients, depending on the limits set for how well a drug needs to perform, to warrant further testing. Sometimes a direct comparison is made between old and new drugs in this phase to more accurately assess whether it is worth going on, but the studies are usually too small to answer the question of whether the new drug is better than the old. The gold standard trial of efficacy which determines whether one treatment is better is the randomized phase three study.

In phase three trials, patients with the cancer of interest are randomly allocated to the old or new treatment. The random allocation ensures that there is no bias in selecting patients as to which treatment they will receive, but more importantly, any unknown factors that could influence outcome that are not due to the treatment given, will be randomly, and therefore hopefully evenly, distributed across the treatment groups in the trial. Often the patients are 'blinded' as to whether they are on the new or old treatment so that there is no bias in their responses, particularly if they have to make subjective assessments of the severity of side effects. These methods mean that the only difference between the treatment groups is the treatment to which they have been allocated and therefore any differences in results will be due to the treatment allocated.

These trials usually require hundreds of patients depending on how small a difference between the treatments is being sought. The difference should be clinically meaningful, that is, an outcome that shows sufficient improvement to warrant its use and not just a small difference such as a couple of weeks of improved survival, which may represent a statistically meaningful difference but will be of little value to a patient. Usually if two randomized trials show superiority of a new treatment it is introduced into routine care. The gold standard endpoint for efficacy is the survival of the patient. However, other considerations such as the toxicity of the treatments also require comparison as there may need to be trade-offs in determining which treatment to use. Even if adopted into clinical practice, the use of the new treatment still needs to be monitored carefully for any longer term side effects. It is also helpful to identify subgroups of patients where the response to the drug varies from the mainstream.

For new drugs that are targeted to the product of a gene known to be responsible for the growth of a tumour, the initial trials need to show that the drug does hit the target and then causes a change in the growth of a cancer. Patients for targeted drugs need to be selected by an initial test to determine whether a particular patient's cancer displays the target (often a mutated or changed gene or what that gene produces). For a treatment meant to stimulate an immune response, an initial test of whether it is effective may be simply to demonstrate that an immune response occurs.

Trials to find agents which cause cancer

When looking at whether a particular agent causes cancer it would not be ethical to do a randomized study, exposing some people to the agent and comparing to those who had not been exposed, and often large populations are needed to establish the cause of an illness. However, there are studies which can observe populations which are used to help discover the causes of an illness such as cancer.

Cohort studies

In a cohort study, a group of people who do not have a disease is followed over a long time to record the risk factors to which they have been exposed. A cohort is simply a group of people who share a common experience such as they all have been exposed to a potential risk factor (like asbestos, a drug, radiation, or they may be people with a similar occupation which determines what they are exposed to). They are compared to another group within the more general population who have not been exposed to the risk factor being studied, but in all other respects are similar to the cohort being studied. The study then records all those who develop the disease. In that way an association may be made between the risk factor and the disease.

These studies can be done prospectively where the exposures are recorded as you follow the people, or retrospectively where records are used to establish past exposures, but this may rely on memories of exposures, which are never as accurate.

This evidence is not as strong as from a randomized study since it may show an association between a risk factor and a disease like cancer but does not definitely show that one causes the other. Often people jump to conclusions when results of these studies are first reported, but more work is needed to establish that the agent in question actually caused the cancer. For example, let's say that you chose a cohort of skywriters to study and found that they had a higher rate of lung cancer than a matched group in the general population. It is tempting to say that there is something about skywriting that causes cancer. However, you may not have recorded, say, their smoking history and it may be the case that for some reason a higher percentage of skywriters smoked than the general population and it was that, and not skywriting, which was responsible for your observation about the association between the two. This type of confounding factor would be ruled out if you were able to do a randomized trial.

Several studies in different places that report the same finding will add to the evidence, but another way of establishing cause is to demonstrate that there is a plausible mechanism for how a potential agent could cause cancer. This often has to be established by laboratory testing. For example, the link between alcohol and cancer has been underpinned by several possible ways that alcohol can cause cancer. Firstly it is converted to a cancer-causing chemical, acetaldehyde, and this is known to damage the genetic material in the cells (DNA) by preventing it repairing itself. Alcohol is also known to increase the levels of the female hormone oestrogen, which increases the risk of breast cancer. Alcohol damages the liver causing cirrhosis, which increases the risk of liver cancer and also alcohol damages the cells in the mouth and throat making it easier for them to absorb cancer-causing chemicals from tobacco. These different mechanisms for alcohol to cause cancer make it more likely that the association between alcohol and cancer is one of cause and effect.

Alternatively, not being able to identify a cause can mean that the jury is still out over whether the agent causes cancer. This is the case when investigating whether the use of mobile phones can cause cancer. We know that ionizing radiation from nuclear weapons or leaking power stations or exposure to radiotherapy can cause cancer by damaging DNA. However, mobile phones emit a different type of electromagnetic non-ionizing radiation. The only known effect of this on human tissue is to heat it, but how that could trigger cancers such as a brain tumour on the side of the head where the phone is held is unknown. Studies in cells, animals, and humans have not been able to show that, at least with use up to 10 years, the radiation from mobile phones causes cancer.

One of the biggest problems with cohort studies is that they take many years to reach a result. Some studies follow people from birth. This raises the issue of having to keep in contact with the subjects over a long period and there are sure to be those who drop out along the way which may compromise the study.

Case–control study

Case–control studies are quicker and often less costly than cohort studies. Here the study group is people with the disease being studied. Therefore a group of people with cancer, the 'cases', are compared with a similar group who do not have cancer, the 'controls', and they are observed for their exposures to the risk factor being studied, examining how often it occurs in each group. For example, you could study a group of patients with lung cancer and those without and determine the tobacco smoking history of both. In fact, it was a large case–control study that initially suggested the link between smoking and lung cancer which a subsequent cohort study confirmed.

The larger the numbers of people recruited to the study, the more accurate it will be, but unlike cohort studies you don't have to wait until sufficient events (e.g. the development of lung cancer) have occurred before you have a result. Case–control studies are therefore better for studying rarer diseases where you may wait a long time for sufficient events to appear in a cohort study. However, they have the same issue of not providing the same level of evidence of causation as randomized studies because of other factors which may confound the results. Study types are shown in Figure 5.1.

Cancer clusters

We want to use the example of cancer clusters to make the point that often a cause of cancer cannot be found. A cancer cluster is a more than expected number of cancers, usually over a limited time, in a group of people from the same location. This is often reported by the public who are usually concerned about exposure to a cancer-causing agent in their environment. It may be promoted by the press and even sensationalized so it is important to know the

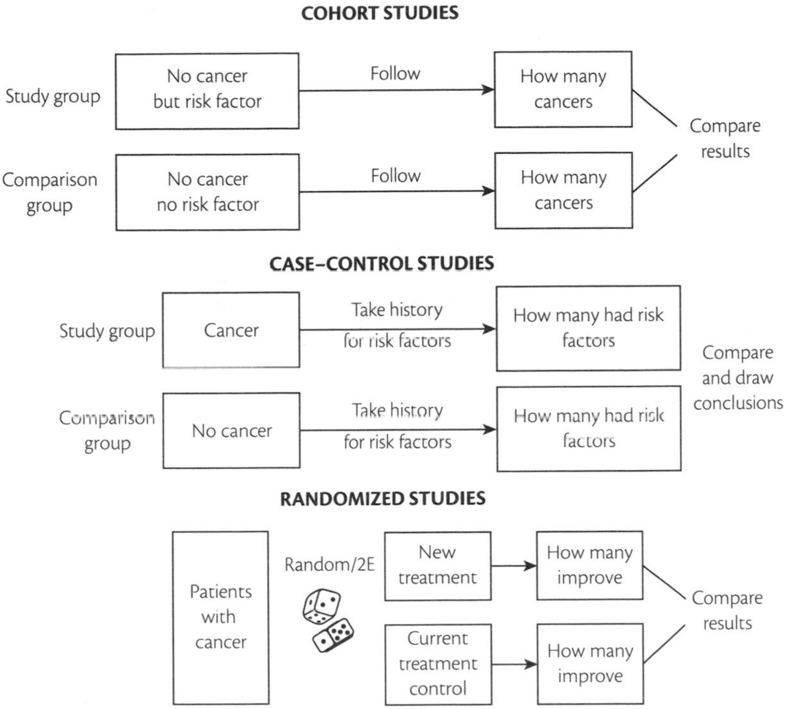

COHORT STUDIES

CASE–CONTROL STUDIES

RANDOMIZED STUDIES

Figure 5.1 Cohort, case–control, and randomized studies.

limitations of investigating such reports. In some situations, a small number of cases may not be outside of the average for the population and so is not a cluster. It is also more convincing if the cancers are all of the same type rather than seemingly unrelated cancers. However, even if there is a true cluster which is a statistically greater number of cancers than expected, most often, even after thorough investigation, no cause is found. Even then the clustering could still have occurred by chance alone.

Sometimes, particularly with rare cancers, the report of a cluster may lead to the discovery of a causative agent. Such was the case with a cluster of angiosarcomas of the liver in a chemical plant which manufactured plastics. On investigation, the causative agent in that plant, and later found in other places, was exposure to vinyl chloride.

Many people may have their pet theories about the causation of clusters. We remember one situation where nurses in a hospital reported a cancer cluster which they attributed to moving into a renovated building where a particular material had been used on the façade. There was no evidence to support that association but the failure to identify another cause led to conspiracy theories about cover-ups. It really just illustrates how difficult it can be to isolate a causative agent out of the large number of potential cancer-causing agents in our environment.

Qualitative research

So far we have looked at research techniques that involve observing, counting, and looking for statistically significant differences between groups (so-called quantitative research). However, if you want to discover why people behave the way they do and how they make lifestyle decisions which may embrace risk factors for cancer, the techniques mentioned earlier will not help. Qualitative research most commonly involves interviews of individuals or groups with the observer interpreting the results. Using the information from particular cases can inform general propositions about which evidence is sought by analysing the data. One technique is to code the transcripts of interviews into segments and then identify similarities and differences between participants in their use of certain phrases that show how they view a particular subject.

Conclusions

We have presented some information about how research is done so that you can make informed responses to reports of trials which purport to show the benefits of a new treatment or headlines about a new risk factor for cancer. It is important to know the limitations of the research that is done and that many studies may be needed before there is sufficient evidence to either change practice and adopt a new treatment, or warn the public about a new risk factor. Often these analyses have been done by major cancer organizations which are known to base their advice on the best available evidence. Websites presenting such information such as those of the National Cancer Institute in the United States, the Medical Research Council in the United Kingdom, or the Cancer Councils in Australia are reliable sources of this information.

Bibliography

American Cancer Society
• http://www.cancer.org/cancer/index

The American Cancer Society is the non-government cancer charity in the United States. It provides a very comprehensive website for the public. It is written so that no specialized knowledge is required to understand it. It provides information on the types of cancer as well as how to prevent and treat cancer. Experts blog on current cancer topics. It also illustrates cancer topics by using stories from people who have had the experience of being diagnosed and treated for cancer. These can often provide hope to people newly diagnosed with cancer.

Cancer Council Australia
• http://www.cancer.org.au/about-cancer/online-resources/iheard.html

This is the iheard website of Cancer Council Australia which was created to answer the many myths, stories, rumours, and exaggerated claims about what causes cancer and how it can be treated. The public are invited to ask any question or paste in the URL of a website that makes a claim about cancer, and an expert will answer the question according to the latest scientific evidence. There are well over 100 questions answered, ranging from whether radiation from microwave ovens causes cancer to whether diets rich in grapes help prevent cancer and it includes often repeated questions such as whether underarm deodorant causes cancer.

Cancer Council Australia: *National Cancer Prevention Policy*
• http://www.cancer.org.au/policy-and-advocacy/prevention-policy/national-cancer-prevention-policy.html

The National Cancer Prevention policy is produced by Cancer Council Australia and is accessed from their website. It is produced by expert committees with members sourced from each of the state Cancer Councils and their supporters. It has been written onto a media wiki platform so that it can be easily updated as new evidence becomes available, and as a web-based document it can be widely disseminated. It has referenced chapters on the preventable risk factors: tobacco control, overweight and obesity, physical inactivity and nutrition, alcohol, ultraviolet radiation, and occupational cancers. Other sections cover screening for breast, cervix, and bowel cancer and discuss screening for high-risk groups in melanoma and case finding for asymptomatic men who want to be tested for prostate cancer, having weighed the risks and benefits. Finally the evidence for the benefits of immunization against the human papilloma virus to prevent cancer of the cervix and hepatitis B to prevent liver cancer is presented.

Cancer Research UK. *Reliable, Easy to Understand Patient Information from Cancer Research UK*
• http://www.cancerresearchuk.org/about-cancer/
Cancer Research UK is an umbrella organization for cancer research in the United Kingdom. As may be expected, the website presents a great deal of information on cancer research and clinical trials in plain English so that patients and relatives can understand their trial options. It gives information on the different types of trials and for those in the region, how they can participate. There is also more general information about cancer types and the drugs used to treat them. A section on coping with cancer not only concentrates on the physical symptoms and side effects of treatment but also the emotional challenges of coping with a diagnosis of cancer. There is also a section of practical aspects of coping including financial issues and the challenges of travel. A forum on the site allows patients to converse with other patients with cancer who face similar issues.

GLOBOCAN 2012. *Estimated Cancer Incidence, Mortality and Prevalence Worldwide in 2012*
• http://globocan.iarc.fr/Default.aspx
GLOBOCAN is the website of the International Agency for Research on Cancer under the World Health Organization. It provides estimates of the number of new cancers each year across the world (incidence), the number of people around the world living with cancer (prevalence), and the number of people dying of the various cancers. This site is regularly updated and its accuracy depends on the sources of the information worldwide, which are, in general, improving. For some countries who do not keep cancer statistics, the rate of cancer is estimated from the countries around them to give a worldwide picture. The website provides sufficient information for researchers and cancer policymakers to be able to perform simple analyses of the data and draw their own graphs to illustrate the statistics.

Mayo Clinic. *Cancer Prevention: 7 Tips to Reduce Your Risk*
• http://www.mayoclinic.org/healthy-living/adult-health/in-depth/
  cancer-prevention/art-20044816
The Mayo Clinic is a world-renowned hospital both for treatment and
research of diseases including cancer. They give good advice to the general
public about how to prevent cancer by presenting tips that people can take
up by modifying their lifestyles to reduce their cancer risk. It is very practical
and goal oriented. There is also access to more detailed publications from
the experts at the Mayo Clinic. They present a multimedia website with text,
images, and videos and they keep their readers up to date with an e-newsletter
covering many topics.

National Cancer Institute
• http://www.cancer.gov/
The website of the National Cancer Institute of the United States of America
is an authoritative source of regularly updated information about all aspects
of cancer. There is information on different types of cancer and on how to
prevent cancer. It provides statistics on how many people get cancer and the
death rate from cancer. This is an excellent website for finding out about cancer research.

NHS Choices. *Preventing Cancer*
• http://www.nhs.uk/LiveWell/preventing-cancer/Pages/Preventing-
  cancer-home.aspx
The National Health Service (NHS) of the United Kingdom Government has
a health website which provides information on a variety of diseases, including
cancer. It also carries advice on cancer prevention. The information is presented using multiple media formats, including video clips. The site emphasizes
healthy choices to enable people to live well. It details health and support services that are available through the British NHS and also has a regular section
for new health news.

World Health Organization. *Cancer Prevention*
• http://www.who.int/cancer/prevention/en/
The cancer prevention section of the World Health Organization (WHO)
website takes a global view of cancer prevention which not only focuses on
personal lifestyle changes including tobacco, obesity, and alcohol but also
includes more external factors including infectious agents and environmental
pollutants as well as occupational cancers and radiation exposure. It shows the
scope of the problems and then the global initiatives that have been devised to
address these aspects of cancer prevention.

Index

Index